BALANCE EXERCISES FOR SENIORS OVER 60

10 Min A Day To Reclaim Your Balance, Prevent Falls And Regain Your Stability

LUNA LIGHT

Disclaimer

This book is intended to provide readers with general information about yoga exercises and routines. The content provided is not a substitute for professional medical advice, diagnosis, or treatment. Engaging in any exercise program carries the risk of injury. While the author and publisher have made every effort to ensure the safety of the exercises and routines described in this book, they cannot guarantee that they are appropriate for every individual. Always seek the advice of a qualified healthcare provider with any questions you may have regarding a medical condition or physical exercise regimen if you are unsure. If you experience pain, dizziness, discomfort, or any other symptoms while performing any of the exercises described in this book, stop immediately and consider seeking medical attention. By voluntarily participating in any of the exercises shown in this publication, you accept the risk of any potential injury.

Contents

SECTION 1: ESSENTIAL KNOWLEDGE

SECTION II: BALANCE EXERCISES

YOUR BONUS VIDEOS

Congrats! Your new book comes with video lessons included.

A lot of time and effort went into making this the best Pilates book and that applies to our videos too. Completed by a certified Pilates instructor, the moves in the videos are correctly done and easy to follow.

Unlike our competitors, you won't have to worry about risking injury, following bad instructions or using improper or dangerous forms with our instructor-certified movements.

HOW TO DOWNLOAD YOUR BONUS VIDEOS:
WRITE AN EMAIL TO:
wall.pilates2@gmail.com

We will reply within a few hours and be sure to write the correct email address, including the "." between "wall" and "pilates".

WE WILL UNLOCK YOUR ACCESS TO THE FULL VIDEO COURSE FOR FREE ONCE YOU EMAIL THE ABOVE ADDRESS.

ALL THE EXERCISES

Warm-up Exercises

Awareness in Movement Exercises

Alignment Exercises

Flexibility Exercises

Strength Exercises

Why I Wrote This Book

"Balance is not something you find, it's something you create."
— Jana Kingsford

It was a warm, sunlit day when my family gathered at our local town park. Our two-mile hikes were a weekly highlight, full of chatter, laughter, and camaraderie. Leading our little group was my beloved Aunt Clara. Her boundless energy and indomitable spirit were an example to all of us.

Little did we know that this day would set the stage for an unforeseen journey that would test our strength and unity. As we strolled along the path, Aunt Clara stumbled and fell. The family rushed to help, but an embarrassed Clara assured us that it was nothing—she'd simply lost her footing.

Fast forward twelve months, and we were back on that same trail. Once again, amazing Aunt Clara was five strides ahead of everyone else. I called out to her to slow down so we younger ones could catch up. That's when it happened …

Aunt Clara took a backward step as if she were going to reverse walk back to us. But suddenly, she collapsed, crumpling to the forest floor like a delicate autumn leaf. I immediately knew that this time it was serious.

By the time I got to her, Aunt Clara was clutching her left wrist and wincing in pain. She'd reflexively tried to break the fall with her left arm and ended up falling on top of it with all her weight.

Within forty minutes, we'd gotten Aunt Clara to the emergency room. X-rays revealed a serious wrist fracture. She also had a nasty cut on her lower left leg that required stitches.

Physical therapy, pain medication, and frustration were now Aunt Clara's realities. The two months she spent off work caused the woman, who a few weeks earlier was the positive energy of the family, to slip into depression.

I was profoundly affected by Aunt Clara's situation. The vibrant woman who once radiated energy was now navigating a world of recovery and healing. I had never realized how debilitating a fall could be for seniors.

I dug into the research and was shocked to discover that falls are one of the leading causes of death in people over the age of 65. It soon became clear to me that the root cause of falls among the elderly is balance issues.

That in itself wasn't a surprise. But the more I researched, the more I found something amazing—for decades, we've been missing a key element in improving balance in seniors …

Strength training for balance.

The stronger your lower body muscles are, the more likely you will be to recover when you stumble, preventing the fall from ever happening.

I discovered that the combination of balance exercises and strength training is the key to becoming confident on your feet.

Hi, my name's Luna, and I'm a personal trainer with a special affinity for working with seniors. Aunt Clara's unfortunate experience ignited my passion to help as many seniors as I can regain the balance and confidence of their youth.

I've personally worked with dozens of people in their 60s, 70s, 80s, and even a few in their 90s. The results of the combination of strength training and balance exercises have been remarkable.

Now, I'm excited to open up the world of balance exercise to you in the pages of this guidebook. It's time to reclaim your balance, regain your confidence, and step confidently into the next chapter of your life.

Let's do this together!

Love,
Luna Light

Who Is This Book For?

If you are concerned about your balance and coordination, then this book is for you. Maybe you're entering your golden years and have been conditioned to think that loss of balance, decreased mobility, and increased susceptibility to a fall are an inevitable part of aging.

It's also possible you're younger and naturally have a bad posture, creating imbalances that cause pain or discomfort in your body. Or maybe you're going through a rehabilitation period for an injury you sustained. I believe this book can and will help you.

When your body is imbalanced, you will continue to add stress in the wrong areas, which will lead to improper posture and pain later down the road. That's why this book will provide a roadmap to countering the natural effects of aging so you can become stronger, more mobile, and more confident on your feet.

Maybe you're a senior who has suffered a fall and lost your balance confidence. This may have led you to adopt the "senior shuffle," to overly rely on mobility aids, or to avoid the mobility-related activities that you used to love. This book will gently guide you through an exercise plan at your level to rebuild your balance confidence and defeat the fear of falling.

Or it could be that you are an active senior who has spent years enjoying various physical activities, but lately, you've noticed a decline in your balance and coordination. It's possible that your fear of falling is also preventing you from doing things you used to love to do. This book is tailored to address the specific needs of active seniors, offering a comprehensive guide to regain and maintain balance, mobility, and confidence.

Or maybe you are a busy senior, juggling family responsibilities and various commitments, struggling to find time for dedicated exercise. This book recognizes seniors' unique challenges and provides practical solutions that seamlessly fit into your schedule. Dedicating just a few minutes each day to targeted exercises can enhance your balance and coordination, contributing to a healthier and more active senior lifestyle.

Regardless of your specific situation, this book is designed with seniors and anyone going through rehabilitation in mind, offering a roadmap to counter the natural effects of aging and promoting a fulfilling and active life no matter what age you are!

Your Free Gift

Congrats! Your book comes with a bonus:

The Ultimate Kegels Guide

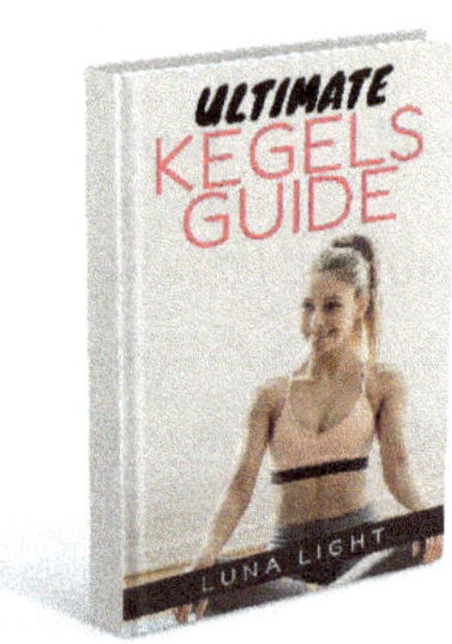

You may have heard of Kegels before... but, unfortunately, there is widespread misinformation about hold time, the number of repetitions, and how to actually perform the contractions that do more bad than good.

When done right, Kegels are a powerful way to build endurance, increase strength in your core, and enhance your sex life. The Kegels exercise we created comes directly from Tim Sawyer, a top physical therapist who worked with doctors at Stanford University[1] to develop rehabilitation programs.

This exact Kegels exercise has helped tremendously in improving my pelvic floor tone, enhancing my sex life, and developing a strong core.

All you have to do is go to wallpilates.org to download it for free. Alternatively, scan the QR code below:

---

[1] Dr. Wise and Dr. Anderson authored A Headache in the Pelvis: A New Understanding and Treatment for Chronic Pelvic Pain Syndromes and consulted Tim as the main physical therapist for their treatments.

How to Use This Book

As a personal trainer, my passion is to work one-on-one with seniors who want to improve their balance, regain their confidence and independence, and get back the vitality of their youth. My goal in writing this book has been to make you feel as if I'm right alongside you, guiding you as you become increasingly confident with your balance and mobility.

As a result, I've made this guide as user-friendly as I know how. There are two main sections in this book:

- Essential Knowledge

- The Exercises

In the Essential Knowledge section, we'll expose the myth that limited mobility and unsteadiness on your feet are an inevitable part of the aging process. In the process, we'll unpack just what balance is and highlight the three key processes that must be addressed to improve it.

The vital link between strength and balance will also be uncovered. You'll discover how strengthening your lower body muscles is the key to preventing falls and becoming more confident on your feet.

We'll also explore the importance of good posture and how, by incorporating principles from the Alexander technique into your daily life, you can refine your posture, reduce muscular tension, and ultimately enhance your overall sense of balance and well-being.

The Exercise section has five parts, as follows:

1. **Warm-Up:** These gentle movements will activate your muscles, get the blood flowing, and promote joint lubrication.

2. **Awareness in Movement:** These exercises increase the intensity and range of the exercises, placing more stress on your muscles and getting your heart rate up slightly. They introduce mobility, balance, and bodily awareness.

3. **Alignment:** These moves are designed to increase your heart rate as they engage specific muscles through a full range of movement.

4. **Flexibility:** These exercises improve joint flexibility and muscle elasticity, enabling you to react more effectively during body position changes.

5. **Strength:** These exercises promote balance, stability, and overall functionality.

Your customized workout program will involve exercises from each section, done in the following order:

- Choose 3 warm-up exercises to begin your workout.

- Choose 3 exercises from the awareness in movement section.

- Choose 3 exercises from the alignment section.

- Choose 3 exercises from the flexibility section.

- Choose 3 exercises from the strength section.

Follow this program for 2 weeks. Then, vary your workout every 2 weeks by choosing new exercises. This will keep your workout interesting and full of variety while you gain strength and balance in your whole body.

SECTION 1:
ESSENTIAL KNOWLEDGE

What is Balance?

"Balance in the body is the foundation for balance in life."
— B.K.S. Iyengar

Balance is the body's ability to remain stable and in control, whether stationary or mobile. To achieve balance, a range of bodily systems seamlessly work together to keep us upright and steady.

Balance involves a coordinated interplay of the following bodily processes:

Vestibular System: The inner ear contains structures responsible for detecting head position and movement changes. This information is sent to the brain, where it is interpreted to help determine spatial orientation. Movement adjustments can then be made to maintain balance.

Proprioception: This is the body's ability to sense its position in space. Our muscles and joints contain proprioceptors, which signal the body's position to the brain. The brain then directs real-time adjustments to maintain balance.

Vision: The eyes provide information about the environment and its relationship to the body. This visual input is particularly important when other sensory cues are compromised.

Muscular Strength and Coordination: Strong and coordinated muscles, especially those in the core and lower body, are essential for maintaining balance. These muscles work together to support the body's weight and respond to changes in position.

Practically, balance comes down to the interplay of four bodily actions:

1. Posture
2. Flexibility
3. Stability
4. Mobility

Posture: Poor posture is a major contributor to balance problems. When your body's segments are not properly aligned, stress is applied to your muscles and joints. When your posture is corrected, the realigned body properly distributes your body weight, improves your center of gravity, and enhances your overall stability.

Flexibility: A flexible person is able to move their muscles and joints through a full range of motion. This is vital for adaptive and fluid movement. A flexible body can also make quick-fire adjustments to avoid a tumble when walking on unstable terrain.

Stability: A stable body can resist movement or maintain control in the face of external forces. A stable base gives you a foundation for dynamic movements to prevent swaying or tipping over. Boosting the stability of your core, hips, and lower body is especially important to enhance balance.

Mobility: A mobile body can move freely and easily. It can adapt to different conditions, adjust to changes in terrain, and respond to external stimuli. Balance requires a balance between stability and mobility. For example, mobile ankles and hips allow for smoother weight shifts during walking, contributing to overall balance.

How Aging Affects Balance

Balance is not an innate ability; infants lack balance in their early months but gradually develop it between four and six months as they learn to coordinate muscles through crawling, walking, and running.

As the child becomes a young adult, their balance and coordination improve, enabling activities like skateboarding and dancing. However, from about the age of 40, age-related changes begin to impact balance.

Here's an overview:

- **Bone Density Changes:** After the fourth decade, bone density decreases, causing bones to shrink and become more prone to fractures.

- **Muscle Changes:** Aging leads to a decline in muscle mass, particularly in fast-twitch fibers responsible for quick movements, affecting reflex abilities.

  Sarcopenia, or age-related muscle decline, results in lower body weakness, contributing to falls among seniors.

- **Hormonal Changes:** Testosterone, vital for muscle building, declines by about one percent per decade from age 30, contributing to sarcopenia.

  Lower levels of estrogen in women accelerate age-related bone loss, increasing the risk of fall injuries.

  Diminished hormone sensitivity further reduces effectiveness, impacting overall health.

- **Brain & Nervous System Changes:** Brain shrinkage begins around age 40, affecting the prefrontal cortex, cerebellum, and hippocampus.

  Neurons gradually shrink, retract dendrites, and produce fewer synapses, leading to slowed reflexes, balance issues, and memory lapses.

- **Body Composition Changes:** Age-related muscle loss is accompanied by increased body fat due to a slowing metabolism. Metabolism decreases annually after age 30, resulting in a caloric excess stored as body fat, leading to weight gain.

  Weight gain contributes to balance problems by adversely altering a person's center of gravity, increasing joint stress, decreasing flexibility and range of motion, and negatively affecting proprioception.

In the following chapters, we're going to explore the psychological and lifestyle effects of losing your balance, and I'm going to show you in the 2nd section how to regain your balance using the 4 pillars in our exercise program:

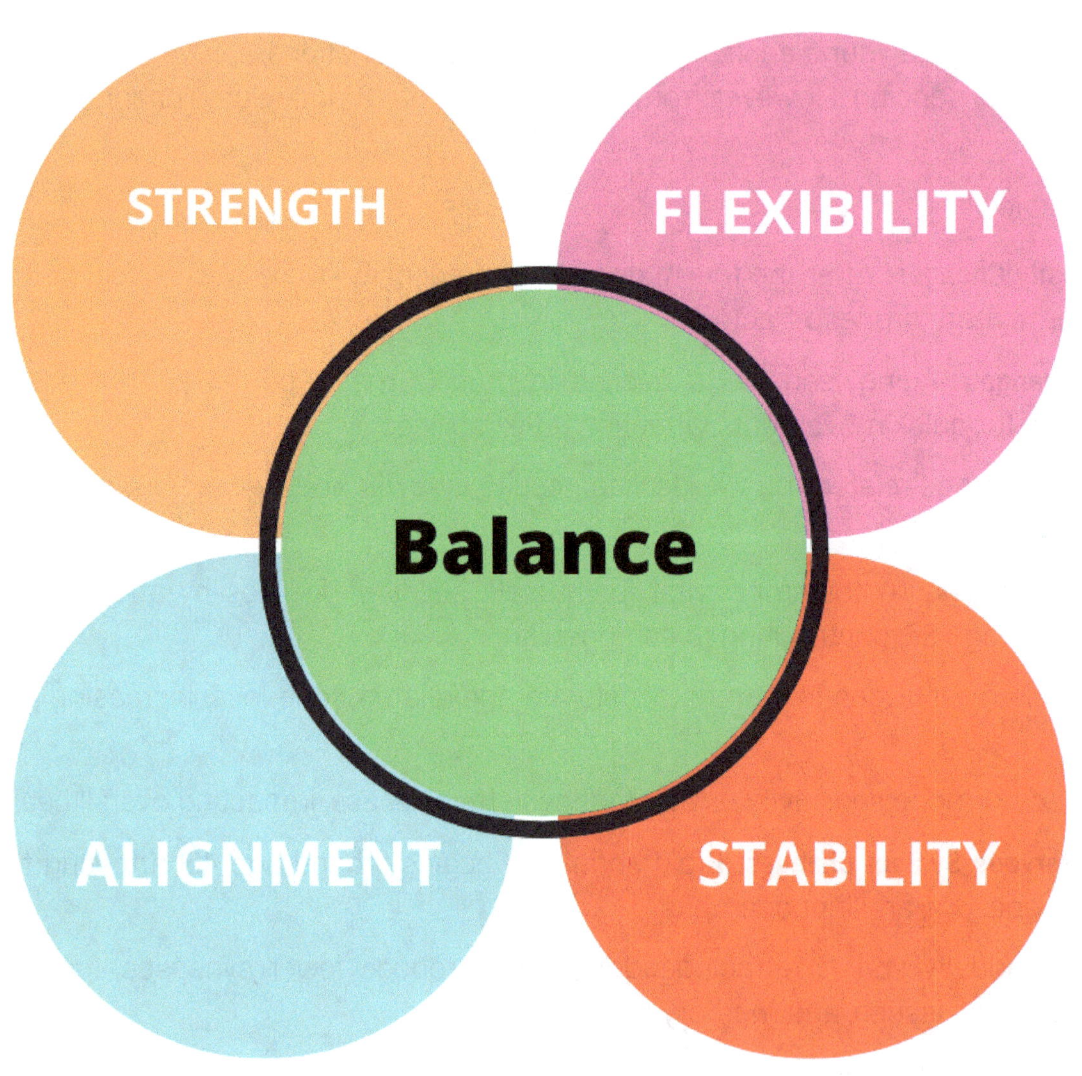
STRENGTH
FLEXIBILITY
Balance
ALIGNMENT
STABILITY

The Psychological Effects of Balance Loss

It wasn't until my Aunt Clara's fall that I realized how the repercussions of a loss of balance can affect a person's mental health. I stood by and watched a formerly vibrant, optimistic, upbeat motivator slide into negativity, frustration, and a lack of confidence.

Here's how impaired balance can affect your psychological health:

Lack of Confidence: The fear of falling can cause a person to avoid activities they once enjoyed, including going out in public. This can lead to a sense of isolation and withdrawal.

Anxiety and Fear: Folks with balance challenges may become extremely anxious about suffering a fall. This can negatively affect their stress level and overall health, leading to increased blood pressure and pulse rate and contributing to social isolation.

Depression: Constantly struggling with balance can cause feelings of helplessness, dependence, and frustration. This may contribute to depression as seniors see their independence slipping away.

Reduced Quality of Life: Battling with balance every minute of every day can significantly impact a person's quality of life. The person's sense of purpose, happiness, and fulfillment can all be diminished.

Cognitive Impact: The daily balance challenge can be mentally exhausting. This can cause mental fatigue, making concentrating and processing information difficult.

Social Isolation: A senior with balance problems may be inclined to avoid social situations because they don't want to be labeled as slow or unsteady. This can contribute to feelings of loneliness.

Social Issues Associated with Balance Problems:

- Seniors may feel self-conscious about their perceived slowness, especially in group settings, elevators, or while waiting in lines.

- Using public transportation can become a source of stress as seniors fear inconveniencing others with their slower pace.

- Seniors may avoid social gatherings or decline invitations due to concerns about their mobility.

- Seniors may fear becoming a burden on others, especially if they require assistance due to balance issues.

The Strength/Balance Connection

The stronger your muscles are, the more functionally able you will be. So, a 75-year-old woman who works to strengthen her quadriceps and glutes will have better balance than one who does not. The problem is that we start losing strength and muscle tissue consistently from about the age of 30. The loss rate is 3–8 percent of your muscle mass every decade from age 30 onward.

This muscle and strength loss, known as sarcopenia, is a major contributor to age-related loss of balance. But it is not inevitable. Strength training has an amazing capacity to reverse the effects of sarcopenia.

I know this from my own practice. I work with many seniors who have steadily lost their muscle mass and strength over the years. Most of them are able to restore a decade's loss of strength in as little as six months. In a year, they're as strong as they were twenty years previously.

This increased strength profoundly affects these people's confidence level and dramatically improves their balance. They are now better equipped to react when they find themselves slipping or falling.

Their quadriceps, glutes, hamstrings, and calves are able to create a stable base that allows them to stay on their feet rather than crumple to the floor.

Their type 2 muscle fibers create a counterbalance to work against the pull of gravity and keep them upright. And their strong core provides essential support, enhancing overall stability and posture.

Strength training has advantages that go beyond increasing muscular mass. It stimulates the production of hormones that aid in muscle growth and repair. Additionally, increased muscle mass can positively impact metabolism, bone density, and joint health.

The Deep Core Connection

The muscles that make up your deep core play an essential part in keeping you steady on your feet. These innermost muscles at the center of your body contribute to stability and support. These are:

Transverse Abdominis

Situated as the innermost layer among abdominal muscles, the transverse abdominis (TrA) acts like an internal weight belt. Contraction of the TrA produces hoop tension, resembling a girdle or corset around the midsection. A weakened TrA fails to cinch tightly, leading to spinal and pelvic instability. This can cause lower back or hip discomfort due to an increased load on these regions.

Multifidus

Positioned along the spine across three joint segments, the multifidus plays a crucial role in providing stability at each segmental level.

Pelvic Floor

The pelvic floor muscles form a hammock-like structure extending from the pubic bone to the hip bone. These muscles offer protection to vital organs such as the uterus, bowels, and bladder in women, and the bladder and bowels in men.

Diaphragm

Serving as the muscular partition between the chest and abdominal cavities, the diaphragm works with the pelvic floor and transverse abdominis to provide stability and support to the core.

Balance Check

Let's start with a quick balance check. Because without stability, bad form can cause injuries and repetitive stress to your whole body. That's why we want to perform all the exercises in a stable manner. As you gain stability, everything you do will feel more balanced. We'll call this "balance awareness."

The first step in balance awareness is your feet.

Balance Check Instructions

1. Stand straight in front of a mirror facing the wall.
2. Feel the alignment of both your feet. Are they properly aligned, or is one foot in front of the other? Are your toes pointed forward with a slight outward tilt? This is the natural alignment of the feet:

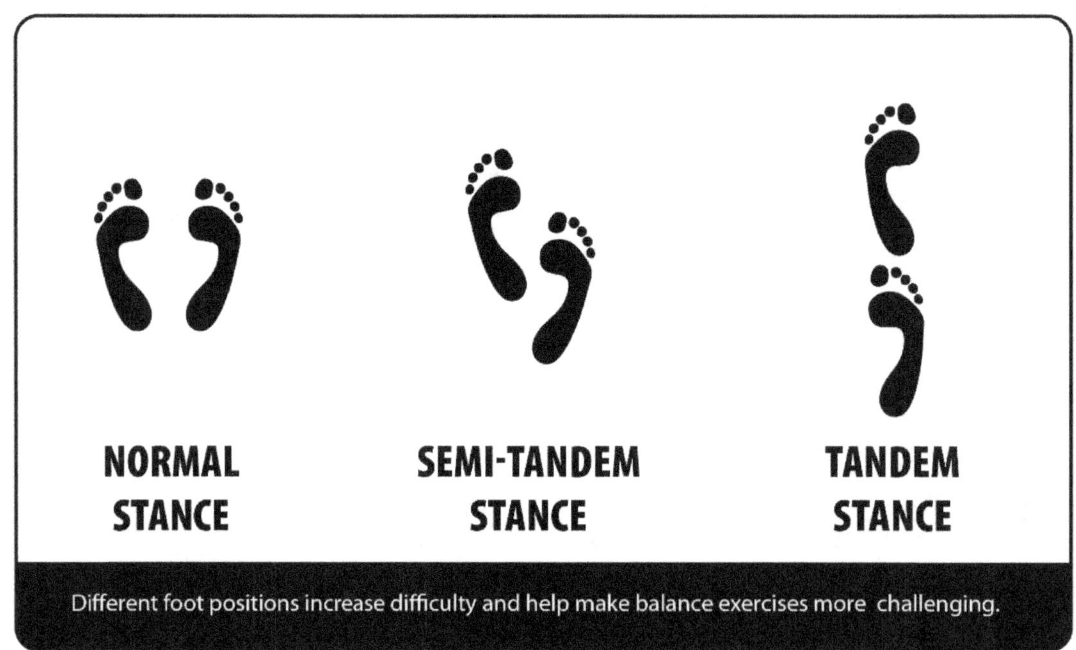

3. Now, feel the weight of your body on your feet. Where is the point of center? Is it toward your toes? Or are you always "on your heels?" Or always "tip-toeing" around? The center of weight should be toward the center of your foot, straight down from the ankles.
4. Stop here, take a breath, and feel your weight distribution—it should be balanced fifty-fifty on both feet. Imagine your spine passing down toward your knees and down to your ankles. The image below shows all the alignments you can build awareness around: the head controlled by the neck, the shoulders, the core and hips, your knees, and your feet.

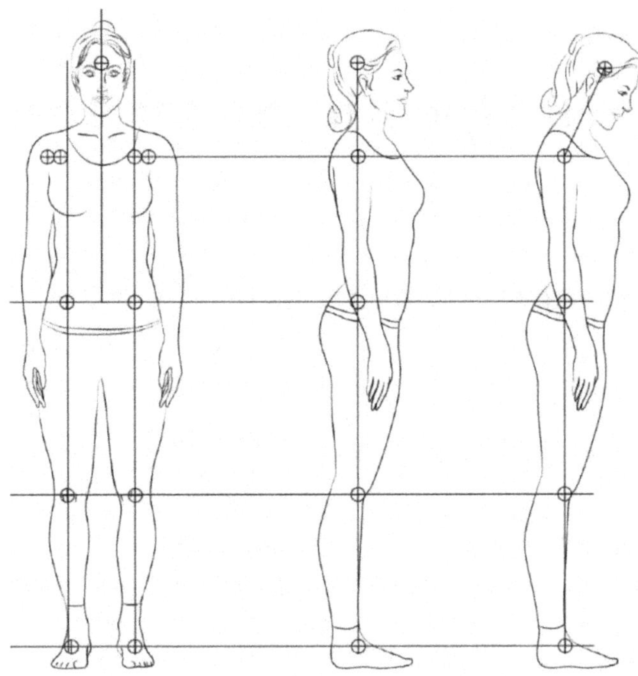

5. Use a mirror and look directly at your alignment from head to toe. Turn sideways and look now. How does your body feel? With your face forward, feel the weight distribution on your feet. Take three breaths here and just feel your body. Imagine a smooth line that goes from the top of your head down your spine and through your feet into the ground. Here are some examples of common dysfunctions:

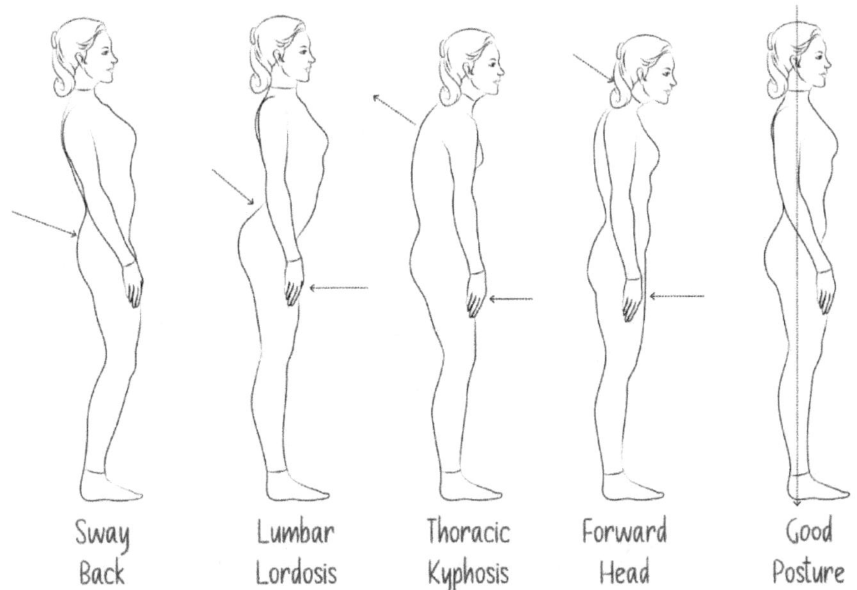

Don't worry about getting it 100 percent right. Just being aware of this will increase your ability to correct any postural issues over time. This exercise trains your mind to become aware of your body's alignment as you go about your day.

Posture and the Alexander Technique

The Alexander technique is a therapy designed to relieve tension and promote balance, good posture, and coordination in everyday activities. Its founder, Frederick Matthias Alexander, discovered that tensions throughout the body are often the cause of many common ailments.

The Alexander technique involves examining posture, breathing, balance, and coordination. As we age, we begin the process of tensing our muscles in response to life's problems. This negatively affects posture. Our shoulders become permanently hunched, our necks become stiffer, and we get into the habit of either sitting in a slouched position or holding ourselves in an artificially rigid position.

There are three stages to learning the Alexander technique:

1. The release of unwanted tension.
2. Learning new ways to move, stand, and sit that minimize tension and bodily stress.
3. Learning new ways of reacting physically, emotionally, and mentally to life's situations.

Releasing Tension

In this initial stage, the focus is on identifying and releasing unwanted tension throughout the body, such as the neck, shoulders, and back. Through gentle and deliberate movements, you learn to release this tension consciously.

Here are three sample movements to target the key tension areas:

Neck Release Exercise:

- Sit comfortably on a chair with your feet flat on the floor and your hands resting on your thighs.

- Gently nod your head forward and backward in a slow, deliberate motion.

- As you nod forward, allow the back of your neck to lengthen, imagining a gentle upward direction.

- As you nod backward, maintain the length in the back of your neck while keeping the movement smooth and controlled.

- Continue this nodding motion, focusing on the release of tension in the neck and encouraging a sense of lightness.

Shoulder and Upper Back Release:

- Stand with your feet hip-width apart and your arms hanging naturally by your sides.

- Inhale deeply, lifting your shoulders toward your ears without any unnecessary tension.

- Exhale slowly, allowing the shoulders to release and drop naturally.

- Roll your shoulders backward in a circular motion, avoiding any unnecessary tightening.
- Repeat this shoulder roll, paying attention to the sensation of releasing tension in the upper back and shoulders.

Spine Lengthening and Release:

- Sit or stand comfortably with an elongated spine, imagining a gentle upward lengthening from the base of your spine to the top of your head.
- As you inhale, focus on expanding the space between each vertebra, creating a sense of length along the spine.
- Exhale, maintaining the elongated spine, and allow any unnecessary tension to release.
- Repeat this breathing and lengthening exercise, gradually releasing tension throughout the entire spine.

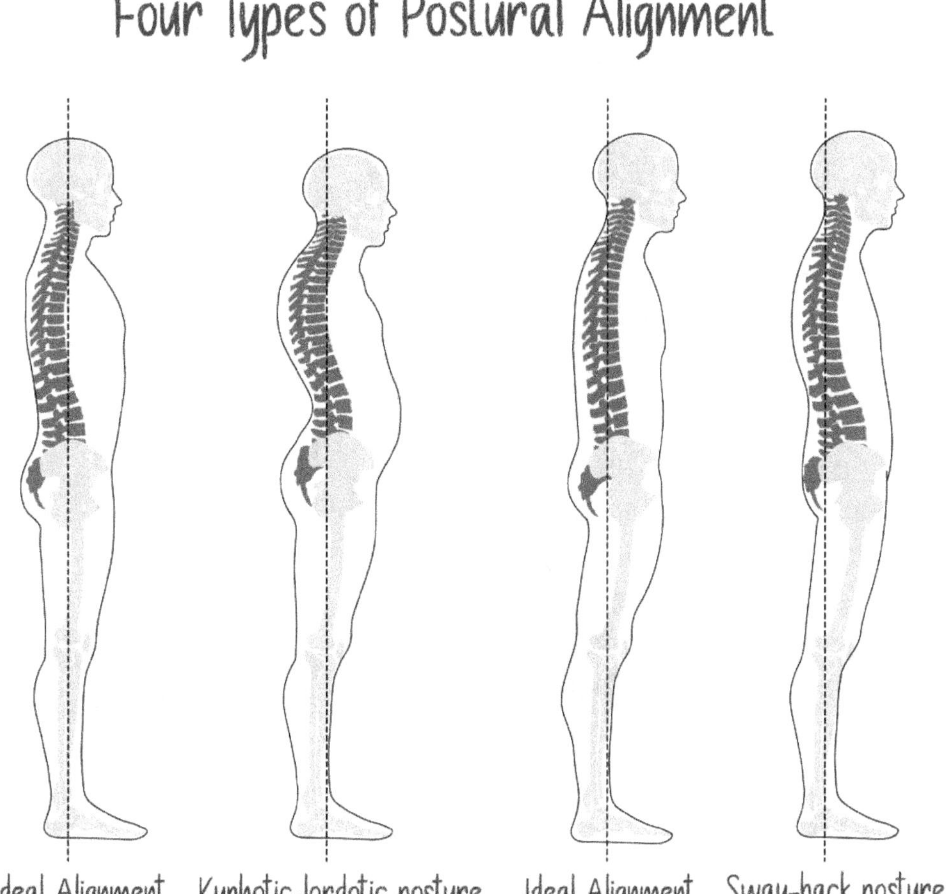

As you practice this awareness, you will begin to develop a taller, more balanced posture. You can use the mirror to check your alignment, from your head to the neck, down the spine all the way to the distribution of weight on your feet. It's all connected!

New Ways to Move, Stand, and Sit

This stage involves exploring alternative ways of sitting, standing, and moving that minimize stress on the body. This includes understanding the principles of alignment, balance, and coordination to foster a more integrated and efficient use of the body. Through guided sessions and practice, individuals cultivate habits that promote good posture and fluid, controlled movements in their daily activities.

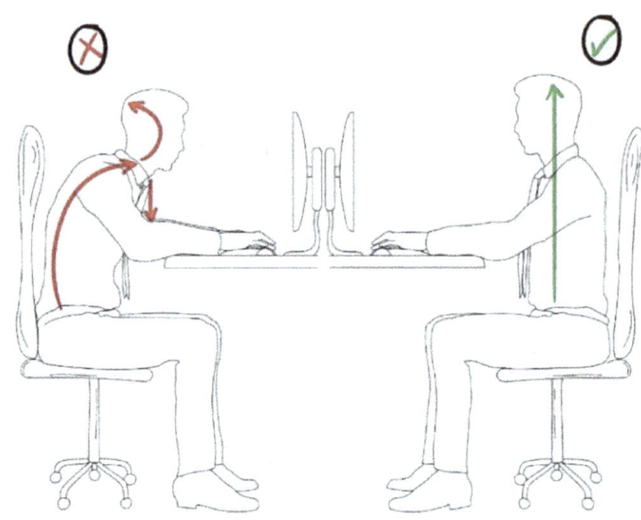

Here are three exercises to promote improved sitting, standing, and moving:

Sitting with Spinal Awareness:

1. Sit on a firm chair with your feet flat on the floor, hip-width apart.
2. Place your hands on your thighs, palms facing down.
3. Gently bring your attention to your sit bones. Imagine them widening and making contact evenly with the chair.
4. Lengthen your spine upward, allowing the crown of your head to reach toward the ceiling.
5. Release tension in your neck and shoulders, letting them soften.
6. Maintain a sense of balance and poise as you sit, engaging your core muscles for support.
7. Breathe naturally, expanding your rib cage with each breath.

Balanced Standing Exercise:

1. Stand with your feet hip-width apart, distributing your weight evenly on both feet.
2. Imagine a string pulling you gently upward from the top of your head.
3. Allow your shoulders to relax and drop, avoiding unnecessary tension.
4. Ensure that your knees are soft and not locked, allowing for a slight bend.
5. Bring awareness to the alignment of your ankles, knees, hips, and shoulders.
6. Engage your abdominal muscles slightly to support your lower back.
7. Practice shifting your weight subtly between your feet, feeling a grounded yet dynamic connection to the floor.

8. Breathe naturally.

Mindful Walking Exercise:

1. Begin walking at a slow, deliberate pace.
2. As you take each step, pay attention to the rolling motion of your foot from heel to toe.
3. Maintain an elongated spine and imagine a gentle upward direction from the top of your head.
4. Allow your arms to swing naturally at your sides, keeping your shoulders relaxed.
5. Coordinate your breath with your steps, inhaling and exhaling rhythmically.
6. Practice mindful awareness of your surroundings, maintaining a sense of balance and poise with each step.
7. Gradually increase your pace, ensuring that each movement remains controlled and intentional.

New Ways of Reacting

The final stage of learning the Alexander technique extends beyond physical movements to encompass emotional and mental reactions to life's situations. Participants develop mindfulness and self-awareness to recognize habitual responses that contribute to tension and imbalance.

This stage emphasizes the mind-body connection, fostering a harmonious and balanced approach to various challenges. The Alexander technique becomes a tool for managing stress and adapting to life's demands with greater ease.

6 Reaction Tips

#1: Mindful Body Awareness

- *Practice regular body scans to become aware of areas where tension tends to accumulate, especially during emotional stress.*
- *Use the principles of the Alexander technique to release tension consciously, allowing for a more mindful and relaxed state.*

#2: Breathing Techniques

- *Incorporate mindful breathing exercises into your daily routine.*
- *Focus on deep, diaphragmatic breathing to promote a sense of calm and balance.*
- *Use the breath as a tool to release emotional and mental tension, aligning with the principles of the Alexander technique.*

#3: Pause and Assess

- *Develop the habit of pausing before reacting to challenging situations.*
- *During this pause, check in with your body and notice any areas of tension or discomfort.*

- *Apply Alexander technique principles to release tension and choose a more balanced and conscious response.*

#4: Maintain Poise Under Pressure

- *Practice maintaining physical poise and alignment even during moments of stress or pressure.*
- *Engage the principles of the Alexander technique to prevent unnecessary physical and mental reactions that may contribute to tension.*

#5: Conscious Movement in Daily Activities

- *Extend the Alexander technique principles to your daily activities, bringing conscious awareness to how you move, sit, stand, and walk.*
- *Apply these principles to create a more intentional and mindful approach to routine tasks, promoting mental clarity and emotional balance.*

#6: Self-Reflection and Adaptability

- *Regularly reflect on your emotional and mental responses to various situations.*
- *Identify habitual reactions and, through the principles of the Alexander technique, explore alternatives that promote adaptability and resilience.*
- *Embrace the idea of continuous learning and improvement in how you respond to life's challenges.*

Before You Begin

Getting started on a balance exercise program is a positive step toward your future. However, it's vital that you do so safely and comfortably.

Here are some important guidelines to follow to ensure that your balance fitness journey is a smooth, injury-free experience.

Consult with your healthcare professional: Before starting any new exercise program, especially if you have preexisting health conditions or concerns, consult with your healthcare provider. They can provide personalized advice based on your individual health status.

Create a safe exercise space: Ensure that your workout area is free from tripping hazards, well-lit, and has a stable surface. Ideally, you should have a clear exercise area of at least one square meter (3'3"). You will also need access to a wall for some of the exercises.

Footwear: Some folks prefer to do their balance workout in bare feet. This enhances their sensory experience and provides a sense of freedom. If you would rather wear shoes, ensure they are comfortable and have nonslip soles.

Clothing: Choose loose-fitting, breathable clothing that allows for a full range of motion. This ensures your comfort during exercise. However, it shouldn't be so loose that it gets caught up with your limbs when you are moving.

Stay Hydrated: Drink water before, during, and after your balance exercises. Hydration is crucial for overall health and helps prevent fatigue. I recommend having a water bottle nearby and sipping from it regularly.

Warm-Up: Begin each session with a gentle warm-up. This could include marching in place or light arm circles to increase muscle blood flow.

Cool Down: Conclude your exercises with a few minutes of slow walking or stretching to gradually bring your heart rate back to normal and improve flexibility.

Modify as Needed: It's essential to listen to your body. If an exercise feels uncomfortable or causes pain, modify it to suit your comfort level. Not all exercises are suitable for everyone, and that's perfectly fine.

Hold on to Support: For some exercises, it's perfectly acceptable to hold on to a sturdy piece of furniture or a wall for added support until you feel more confident.

Remember that the goal here is to enhance your balance and stability at your own pace. Following these guidelines will lay the foundations for a safe and enjoyable exercise routine tailored to your needs. Always prioritize your safety and well-being on your journey to improve your balance.

Support Person: For some of you, limited mobility or injuries may require doing your balance workout when another person is nearby. This is a safety precaution just in case you feel lightheaded, topple over, or need extra assistance.

SECTION II:
BALANCE EXERCISES

The Workout Plan

The workout plan is very simple and can be done in less than 10-15 minutes a day.

Phase A

- Choose 3 Warm-up exercises to begin your workout.
- Choose 3 exercises from the Awareness in Movement section.
- Choose 3 exercises from the Alignment section.
- Choose 3 exercises from the Flexibility section.
- Choose 3 exercises from the Strength section.

Phase B

Change this up every 10 days and pick new exercises.

Phase C

After 30 days, you can do all the exercises in order.

Warm-up Exercises

This section's gentle exercises are meant to "wake up" your muscles, allowing them to move through their whole range of motion, while also improving blood flow and lubricating your joints.

A | CHAIR SPINAL TWIST

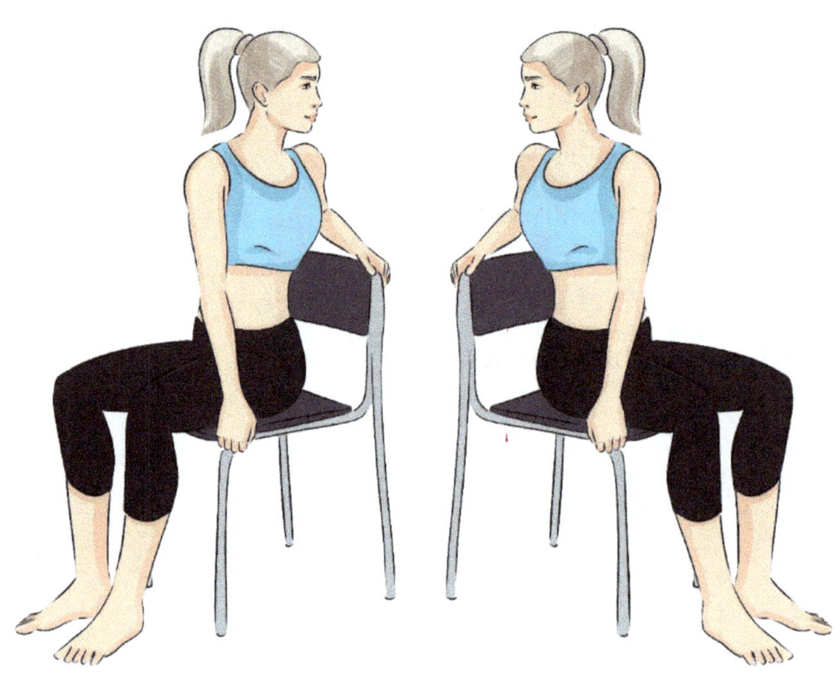

Instructions

1. Sit down on a chair or on the ground with your back straight and your chest up.
2. Place your arm on the backrest of the chair and, as you lengthen your spine, turn backward as far as you comfortably can.
3. Now return to center and turn to the other side.
4. Do 20 reps of 10 on each side.

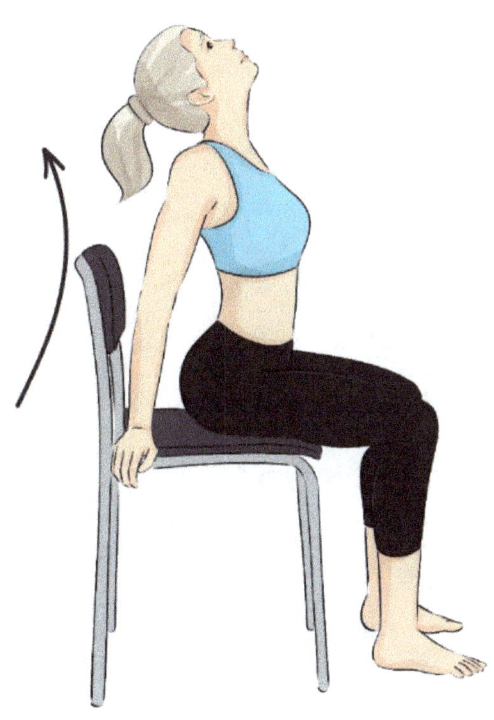

Instructions

1. Sit halfway from the edge and straight up on a chair with your feet flat on the floor. Place your hands behind you firmly on the seat.
2. As you inhale, lengthen your spine and lift your chest. Arch your back and tilt your head upward and backward as far as you can.
3. As you exhale, slowly return to a normal sitting position.
4. Do 10 reps.

Tip

- Don't sit too close to the edge as it's dangerous. Find the center and scoot just enough to place your hands on the chair firmly.

C | CHAIR ARM CIRCLES

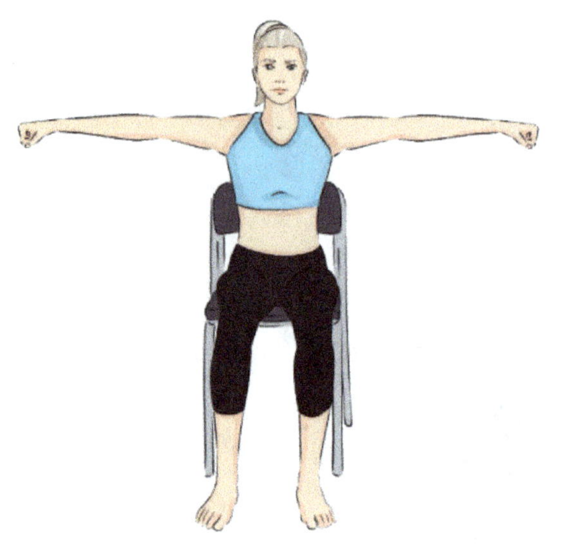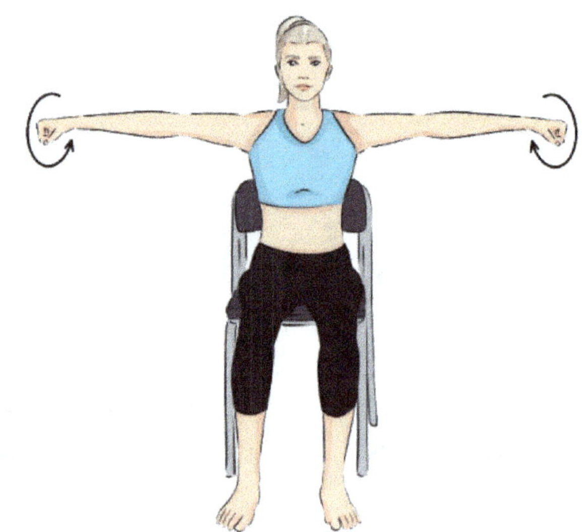

Instructions

1. Sit up straight on a chair with your feet flat on the floor.
2. Extend your arms straight out to the sides, parallel to the floor.
3. Begin making small circular motions with your arms, like you're drawing circles with your hands. You can use an open-handed palm or your fists.
4. Continue the circular motions for 10 seconds.
5. Now, go in the other direction for 10 seconds.

Tips

- Maintain slow and controlled movements to avoid straining your shoulders.
- Gradually increase the size of the circles as you feel comfortable.

D | CHAIR DOWNWARD STRETCH

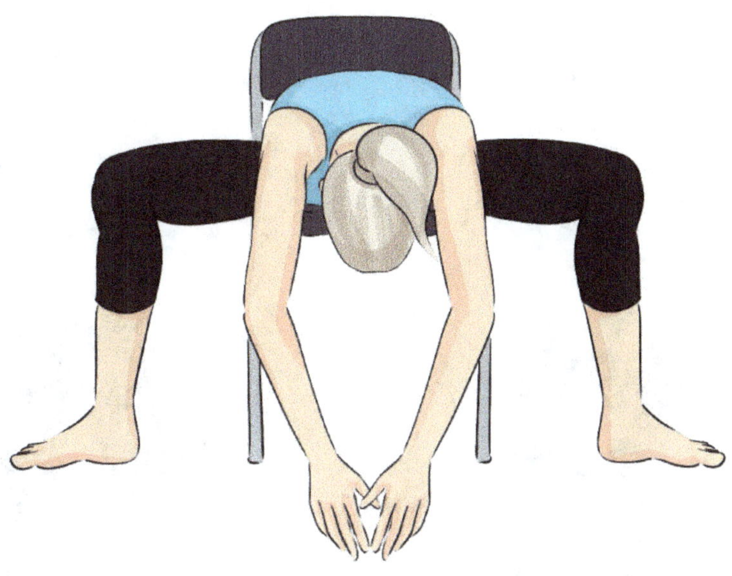

Instructions

1. Sit up straight on a chair with your legs as widely extended as possible.
2. Inhale a deep breath. As you exhale, bend forward with your hands as far down as you can.
3. Repeat 5 times. Each time you extend down, try to go a little further.

Tips

- Avoid sitting too close to the chair's edge.

- If you're super flexible and can touch the ground, see if you can bring your elbows to the ground.

E | HIP CIRCLES

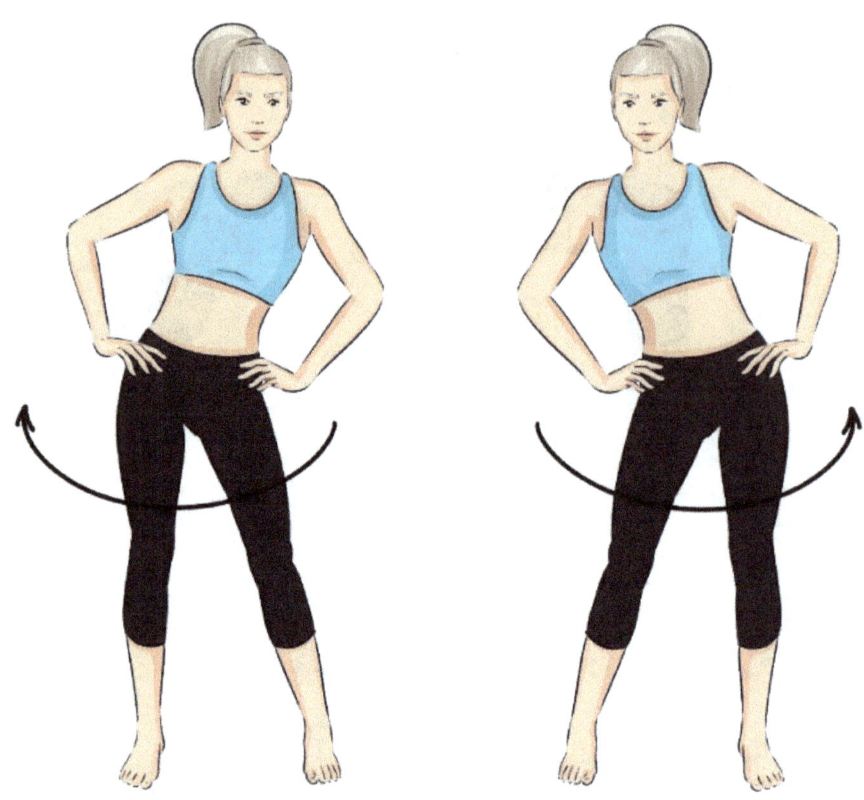

Instructions

1. Stand with your feet hip-width apart and place your hands on your hips.
2. Rotate your hips outward (clockwise), keeping the upper body stable. Circle as far as you can while maintaining stability. Perform 10 circles.
3. Now rotate your hips inward (anticlockwise), keeping the upper body stable. Circle as far as you can while maintaining stability. Perform 10 circles.

Tips

- Breathe steadily throughout the exercise.

- When doing this, feel your hips align with the spine. Do they feel intact or out of place? This is a great exercise to help you sense any posture issues with your hips.

Awareness in Movement

The exercises in this section increase the intensity and range of the exercises, placing more stress on your muscles and getting your heart rate up slightly. They introduce mobility, balance, bodily awareness, and coordination challenge movements.

1 | HEEL TO TOE WALK

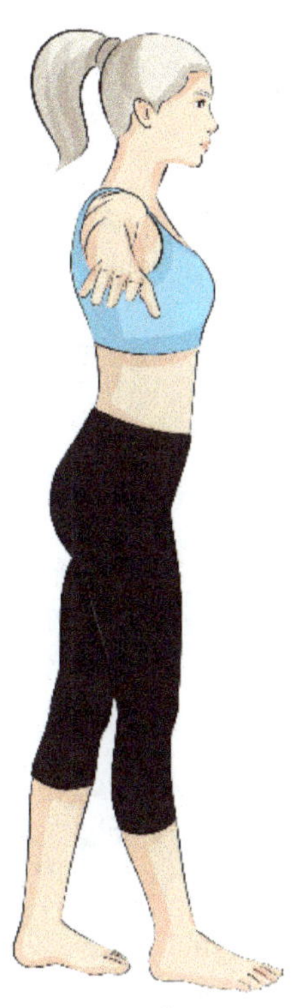

Instructions

1. Stand up straight with your feet together. Ensure your shoulders are relaxed and your gaze is forward. For balance, extend your arms to the sides, keeping them parallel to the ground.
2. Lift your right heel off the floor, keeping your toes on the ground.
3. Place your right heel down directly in front of your left toes so the heel and toes are touching. Your feet should form a straight line.
4. Shift your weight onto the right foot as you bring the left foot forward.
5. Lift your left heel, keeping the toes on the ground.

6. Repeat the process, alternating between your right and left foot. Focus on placing each heel directly in front of the toes of the opposite foot.
7. Continue the heel-to-toe walk for 10 paces. Then turn and do another 10 paces back to the starting point. That represents one set.
8. Complete three sets.

Tips:

- Perform the heel-to-toe walk slowly and with control.

- Concentrate on the connection between your heel and toes with each step.

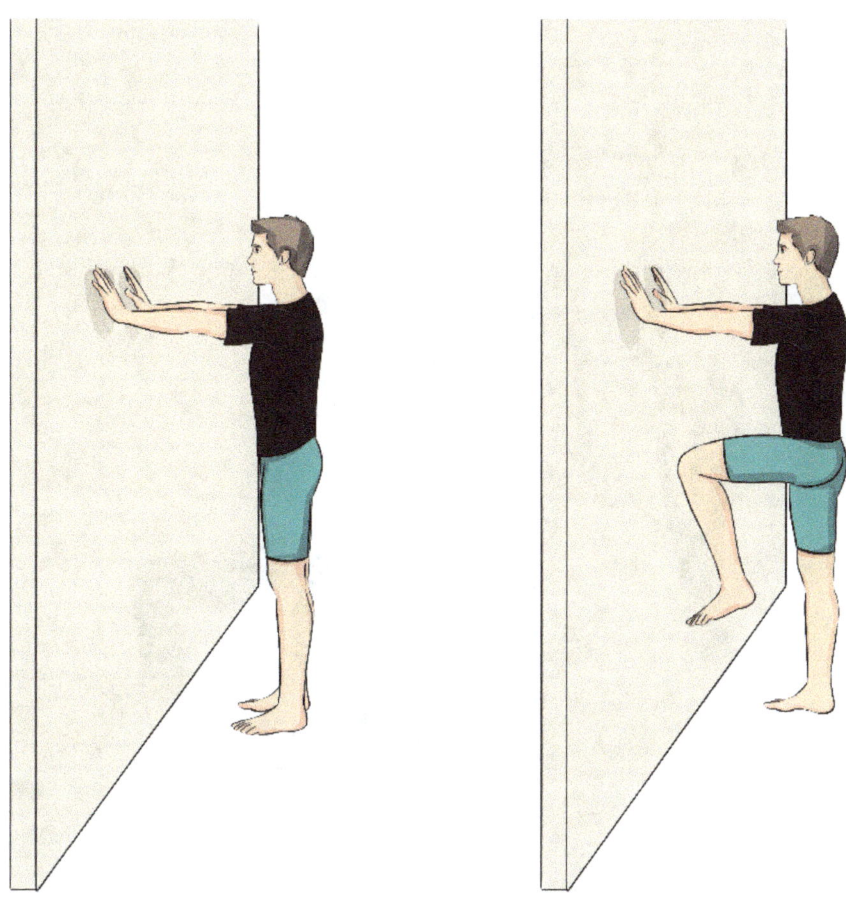

Instructions

1. Stand facing a wall with your feet hip-width apart.
2. Place your hands on the wall at shoulder height, slightly bending your elbows.
3. Lift one foot off the ground, bending the knee at a 90-degree angle.
4. Balancing on the supporting leg, engage your core for stability. Ensure your head, shoulders, and hips are aligned vertically.
5. Focus on a spot on the wall to assist with balance.
6. Aim to hold the lifted position for 15–30 seconds.
7. Keep your supporting knee slightly bent to avoid locking it.
8. Repeat the exercise on the opposite leg.
9. Do 3 sets of 15–30 second holds for each leg.

Tip:

- While balancing, visualize roots extending from your supporting foot into the ground, anchoring you firmly.

3 | WALL LUNGE

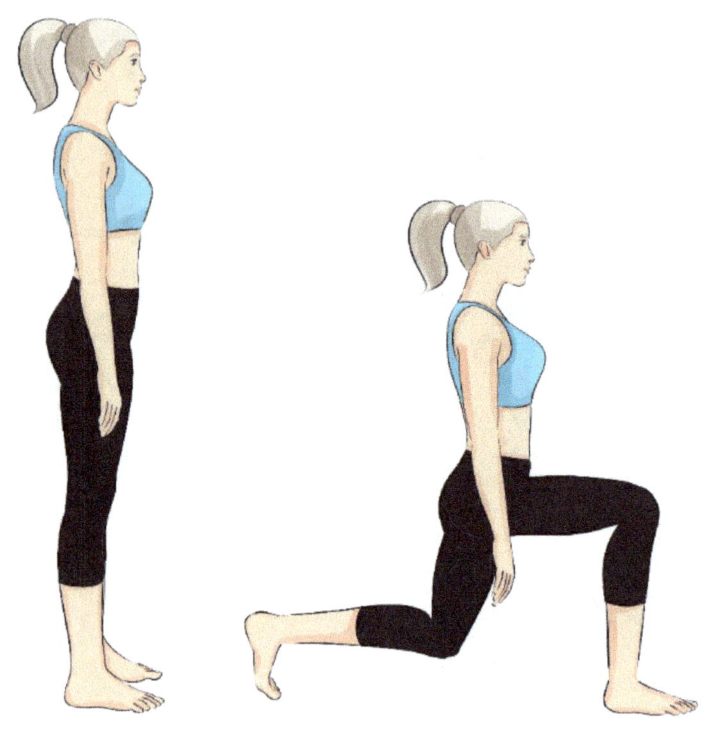

Instructions

1. Stand with your back against a wall.
2. Position your feet about hip-width apart and a step's distance away from the wall.
3. Take a step forward with one foot, maintaining a hip-width distance between your feet. The back foot remains against the wall, heel on the ground.
4. Begin to lower your body by bending both knees. Ensure your front knee is directly above your ankle, forming a 90-degree angle. The back knee gently lowers toward the floor.
5. Keep your back straight against the wall throughout the movement. Engage your core for stability, preventing your lower back from arching.
6. Hold the lunge position for 2−3 seconds, focusing on balance and muscle engagement. Ensure your weight is evenly distributed between the front and back legs.
7. Push through the heel of your front foot to return to the starting position.
8. Repeat the exercise with the opposite leg stepping forward.
9. Perform 3 sets of 12 reps on each leg.

Tip:

- Emphasize proper form rather than trying to achieve a deep lunge initially. Gradually increase the depth of the lunge as your flexibility and strength improve.

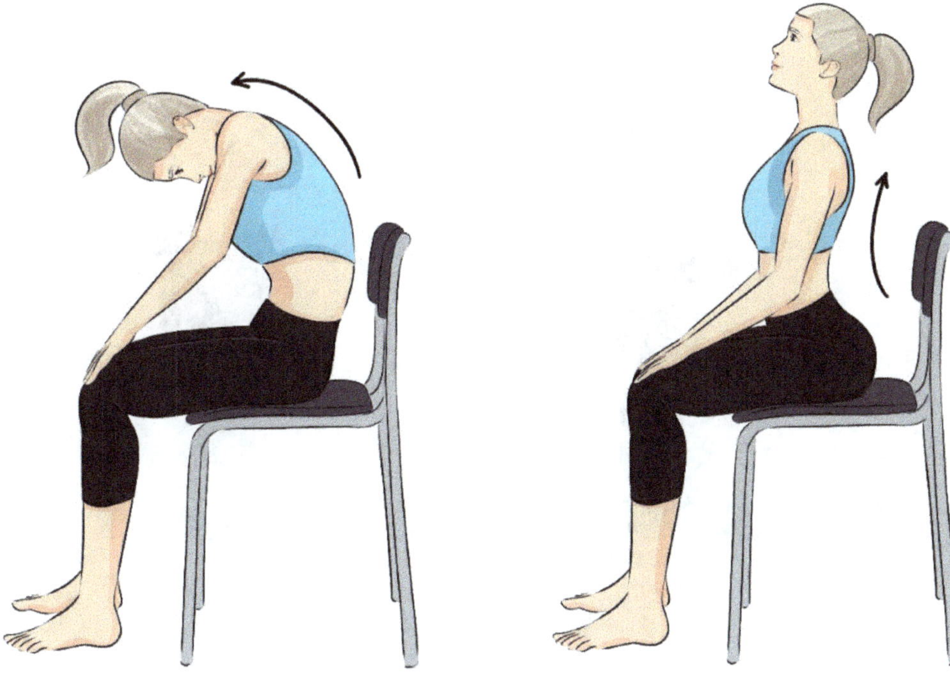

Instructions

1. Sit on a chair with your feet flat on the floor and your back straight. Place your hands on your knees or thighs.
2. Inhale and arch your back, lifting your chest (cow pose).
3. As you exhale, round your back, tuck your chin to your chest, and draw your navel in (cat pose).
4. Continue to flow between cow and cat poses with your breath, inhaling for the cow and exhaling for the cat.
5. Perform this gentle movement for ten reps, feeling the stretch and release in your spine.

Tips:

- You can place your hands on the sides of the chair or hold the armrests for support.

- Keep your movements smooth and controlled, focusing on your breath and the sensations in your back.

5 | BALANCE WALKING

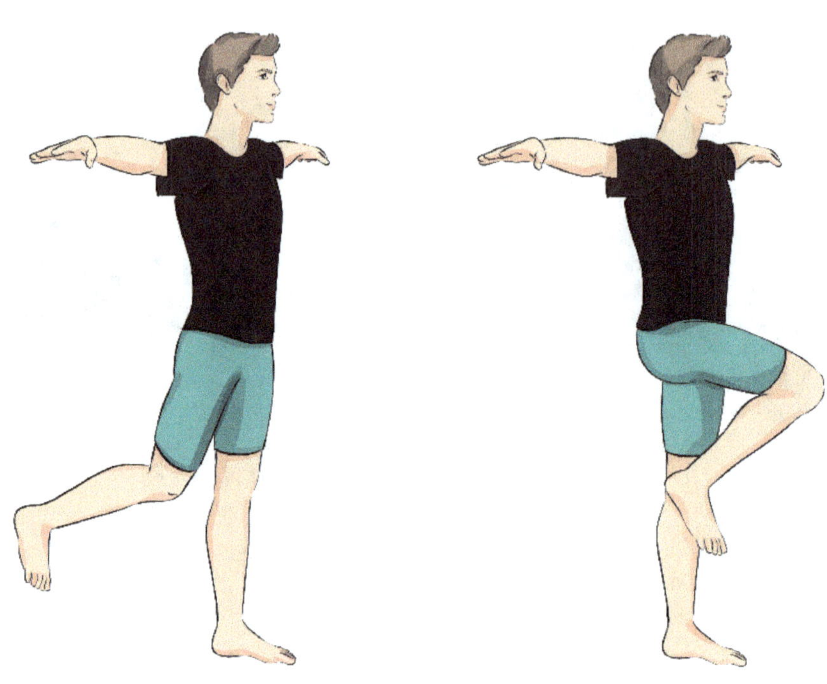

Instructions

1. Stand tall with your feet together and your arms out to the sides for balance. Find a focal point at eye level to help maintain balance.
2. Lift your right foot slightly off the ground, balancing on your left leg. Keep a slight bend in your left knee to engage the muscles.
3. Engage your core muscles and ensure your shoulders are relaxed, not hunched.
4. Take a step forward with your right foot, placing it in front of your left foot. Land heel to toe, rolling through the foot to the ball of the foot.
5. Continue walking in a straight line, placing one foot in front of the other.
6. As you become more comfortable, gradually lengthen your stride. Maintain a slow and deliberate pace to enhance the difficulty.
7. Walk 10 paces forward, then turn around and walk back to the starting point.
8. On the next set, lead with the opposite foot. Complete 3 sets.

Tip:

- This mindful walking enhances the mind-body connection, improving overall balance.

6 | THE GRAPEVINE

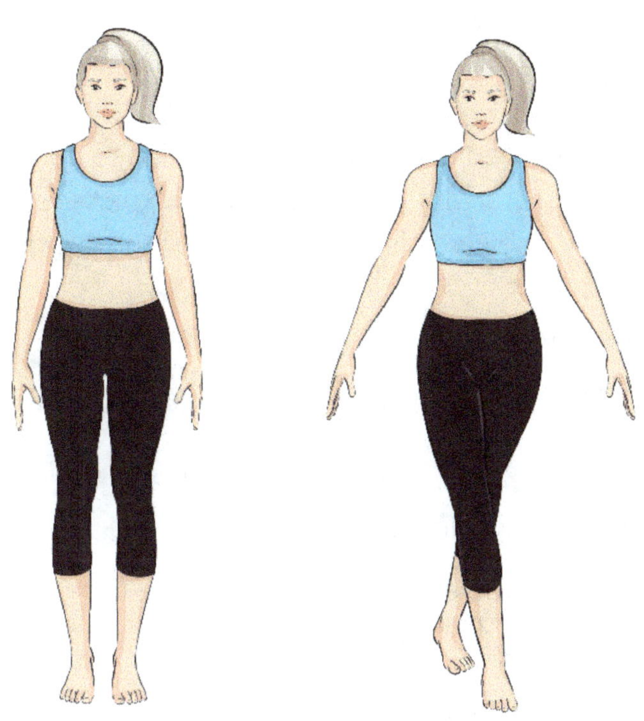

Instructions

1. Stand tall with your feet together and your arms relaxed at your sides. Find a focal point at eye level to help maintain balance.
2. Lift your right foot slightly off the ground, balancing on your left leg.
3. Cross your right foot over your left foot, placing it on the ground.
4. Your right foot should be positioned to the left of your left foot.
5. Take a sidestep to the right with your left foot. Your right foot follows, crossing behind your left foot.
6. Lift your left foot slightly off the ground as you balance on your right leg. Keep a slight bend in your right knee for stability.
7. Cross your left foot over your right foot, placing it on the ground. Your left foot should be positioned to the right of your right foot.
8. Continue the grapevine pattern by side-stepping in alternating directions.
9. Walk 10 paces forward, then turn around and return to the starting point.
10. On the next set, lead with the opposite foot. Complete 3 sets.

Tips:

- Coordinate your arm movements with your leg movements.
- Swing your arms naturally to enhance balance and rhythm.

Alignment Exercises

Alignment refers to the arrangement of body parts in relation to one another. A well-aligned body ensures that the body's center of mass is well-balanced.

Proper postural alignment is fundamental for maintaining balance and stability and reducing the risk of falls, especially in seniors. Seniors with good alignment experience less side-to-side or front-to-back swaying during movement. They are also less prone to stumbling and falling.

Key Elements of Alignment

- Head and Neck: Keep the head in a neutral position, aligning with the spine.
- Spine: Maintain a natural curve, avoiding excessive arching or rounding.
- Shoulders: Keep them relaxed and aligned with the hips.
- Hips: Level hips contribute to a stable base.
- Knees: Slightly bent to absorb shock and provide flexibility.
- Feet: Parallel and hip-width apart for a solid foundation.

7 | PIGEON POSE

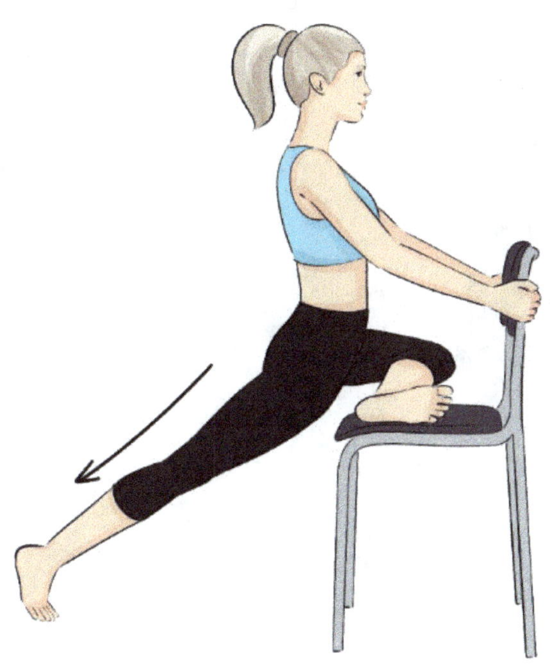

Instructions

1. Stand in front of a chair, facing it. Bend your left leg to place the lower leg on the chair seat, side on.
2. Reach forward to grab the chair's back edges with both hands.
3. Extend your right leg back behind you as far as you comfortably can, resting on the toes.
4. Pull on the chair back as you lengthen your spine and look toward the ceiling.
5. Hold this pose for 15 seconds.
6. Do five reps.

Tip:

*   Focus on engaging your core muscles throughout the pose. This provides stability and enhances the stretch along the sides of your body.

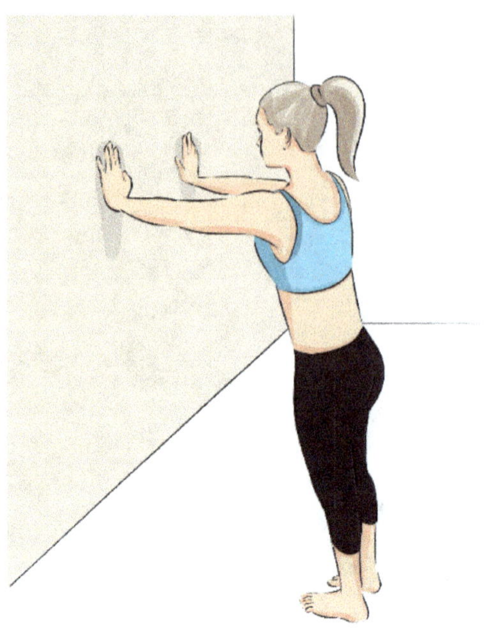 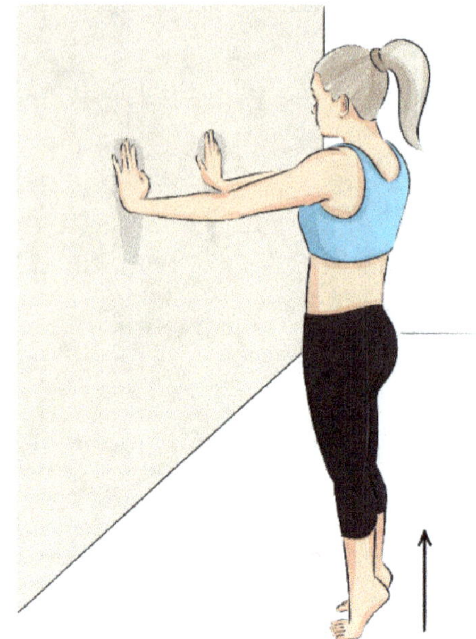

Instructions

1. Stand facing a wall with your feet hip-width apart.
2. Place your hands on the wall at shoulder height for support. Position your feet about a foot away from the wall. Ensure your toes are pointing directly forward. Keep your head, shoulders, and hips in a straight line.
3. Slowly rise onto the balls of your feet, lifting your heels as high as possible. Focus on contracting your calf muscles at the top of the movement.
4. Hold the raised position for a moment, emphasizing the full extension of your calves.
5. Gradually lower your heels back down to the starting position.
6. Perform 3 sets of 15 reps.

Tip:

- To intensify the workout and engage different muscle fibers, try performing the calf raises with one foot at a time. This unilateral approach can help address any strength imbalances between your calves.

9 | GARLAND POSE

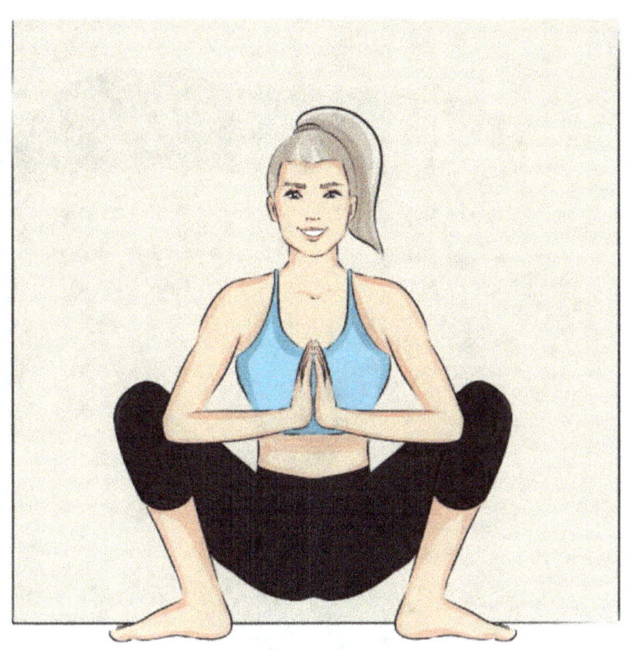

Instructions

1. Stand with your feet slightly wider than hip-width apart and pointing outward at a 45-degree angle.
2. Bend your knees and lower your hips down toward the ground.
3. Bring your palms together in front of your chest, in a prayer position. Use your elbows to gently press your knees apart.
4. Lengthen your spine by lifting your chest. Imagine reaching the crown of your head toward the ceiling. Activate your core by drawing your navel in toward your spine.
5. Stay in the Garland Pose for 30 seconds to 1 minute, or as long as is comfortable for you. Focus on your breath, inhaling and exhaling deeply.
6. To come out of the pose, place your hands on the mat and straighten your legs, coming back to a standing position.
7. Perform 3 sets of 15 reps.

Tips:

- If your heels don't comfortably reach the floor, you can place a folded blanket or yoga block under your heels for support.

- Adjust the width of your stance to find a position that allows you to maintain balance and comfort.

- If you're new to this pose, start with shorter durations and gradually increase the time as your flexibility improves.

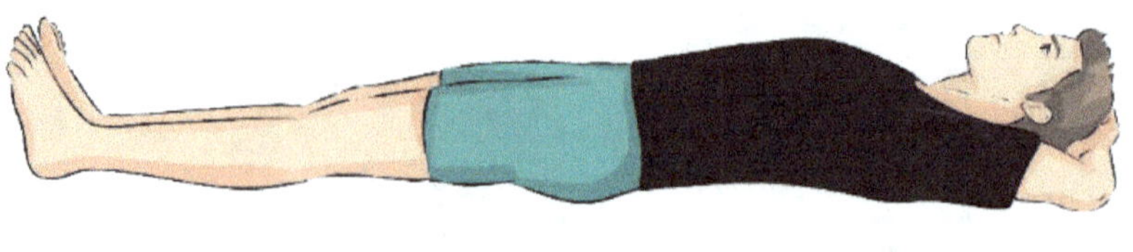

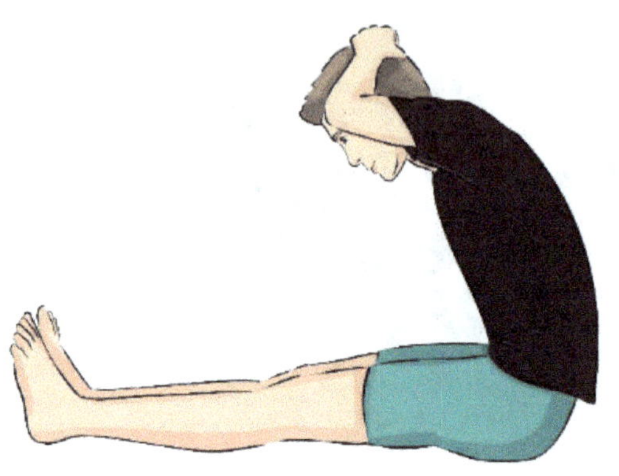

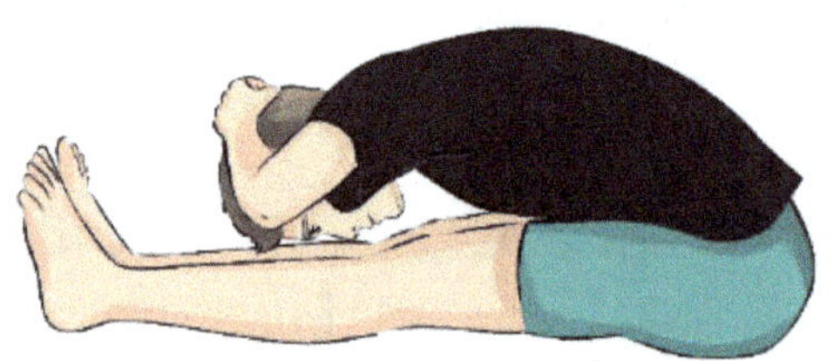

Instructions

1. Lie on your back with your legs extended and your arms reaching overhead. Ensure your legs are together and your arms are next to your ears.
2. Inhale to prepare, and as you exhale, initiate a deep abdominal contraction, pushing your spine into the mat.
3. On the next exhale, lift your legs off the mat to a 45-degree angle. Keep your legs straight and maintain engagement in your abdominals.
4. Continue the exhale and lift your head and shoulders off the mat, reaching your arms toward your toes.
5. Flex your feet, pulling your toes toward your shins.

6. Inhale as you start rolling up through your spine, reaching your fingers toward your toes. Keep your abdominal muscles engaged and maintain the 45-degree angle with your legs.
7. At the top of the movement, you should be in a "C-Curve" position, with your spine forming a smooth curve from your head to your tailbone.
8. Exhale as you slowly roll down through your spine, returning to the starting position with your arms overhead and legs lifted.
9. Repeat 5 times.

Tips:

- Focus on controlled movements.

- Keep your neck long and avoid straining your neck by looking forward or tucking your chin too much.

- Modify the range of motion if needed, especially if you experience any discomfort or strain.

- If you have any neck or back issues, it's advisable to consult with a fitness professional or healthcare provider before attempting the Neck Pull.

Flexibility Exercises

Flexibility is a crucial component of overall fitness, and for seniors, it plays a particularly important role in maintaining balance and preventing falls. Flexibility exercises help maintain and improve joint mobility. As people age, joints can become stiffer, making it challenging to move freely. Improved joint mobility contributes to better balance by allowing a wider range of motion.

Flexibility training enhances muscle elasticity, preventing muscles from becoming tight and rigid. Flexible muscles can respond more effectively to changes in body position and weight distribution, which is essential for maintaining balance.

One of the primary concerns for seniors is the risk of falls. Flexibility training, especially in the lower body muscles and joints, improves the ability to react quickly to unexpected shifts in balance, reducing the likelihood of falls.

11 | WALL ANGEL

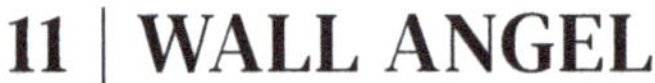

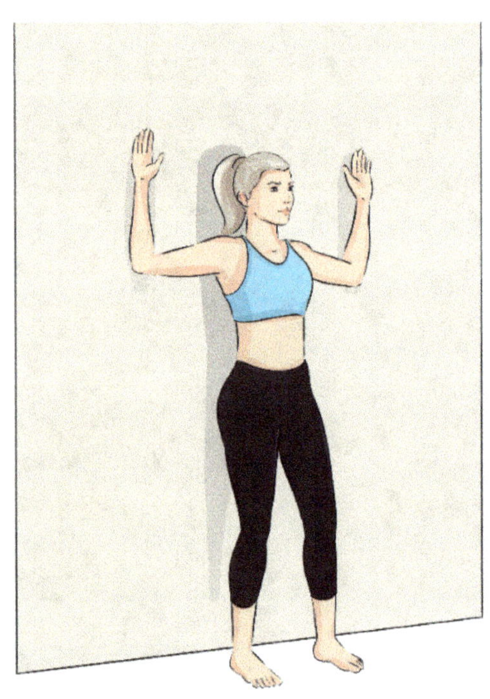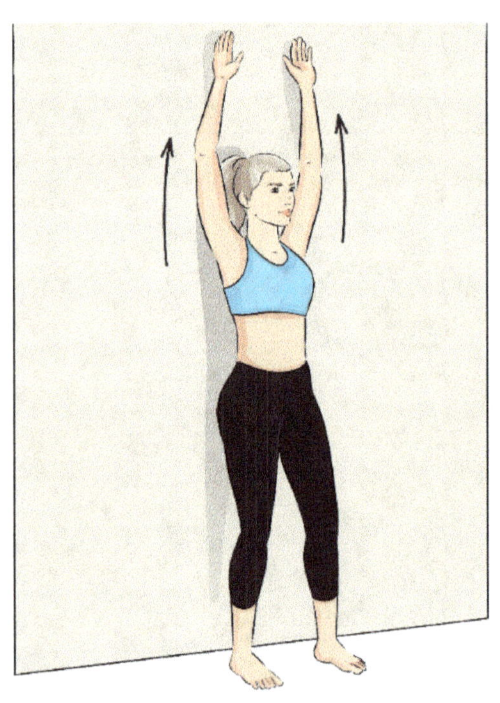

Instructions

1. Stand with your back against a wall. Make sure your feet are about hip-width apart and a few inches away from the wall.
2. Activate your core muscles by drawing your navel in toward your spine. This helps to stabilize your spine and pelvis during the movement.

3. Raise your arms to shoulder height and bend your elbows to create a 90-degree angle. Your palms should be facing forward, and your forearms should be parallel to the ground.
4. Press your entire back, arms, and hands against the wall.
5. Slowly slide your arms upward along the wall, maintaining contact with the wall at all times. Reach as high as you can comfortably without lifting your arms off the wall.
6. Slowly lower your arms back down to the starting position, maintaining contact with the wall. Focus on controlled movement throughout.
7. Perform the Wall Angel for 15 reps.

Tip:

- If you find it challenging to keep your entire back against the wall, especially the lower back, it's okay to have a slight natural curve in your lower back.

12 | LEG SWINGS

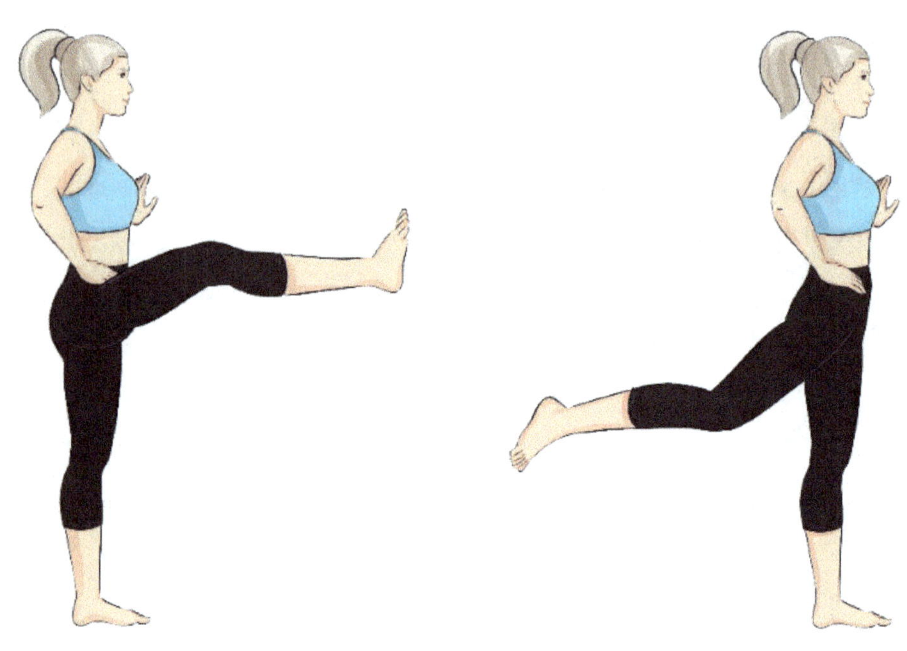

Instructions

1. Stand next to a wall with your feet hip-width apart and your shoulders relaxed. Hold on to the wall with one hand for support. Your arm should be extended at shoulder height.
2. Tighten your core muscles to stabilize your torso and maintain good posture throughout the exercise.
3. Lift one leg in front of you as high as is comfortable, keeping it straight.
4. Swing the leg backward behind you, allowing your hip to hinge.
5. Continue this forward and backward swinging motion for 10–15 swings on each leg.

Tips:

*   Keep your standing leg slightly bent to absorb the swinging motion and avoid locking your knee.

*   Do not force the range of motion; swing your leg within a comfortable and controlled range.

*   If you have any balance concerns, perform the leg swings near a sturdy chair or countertop for additional support.

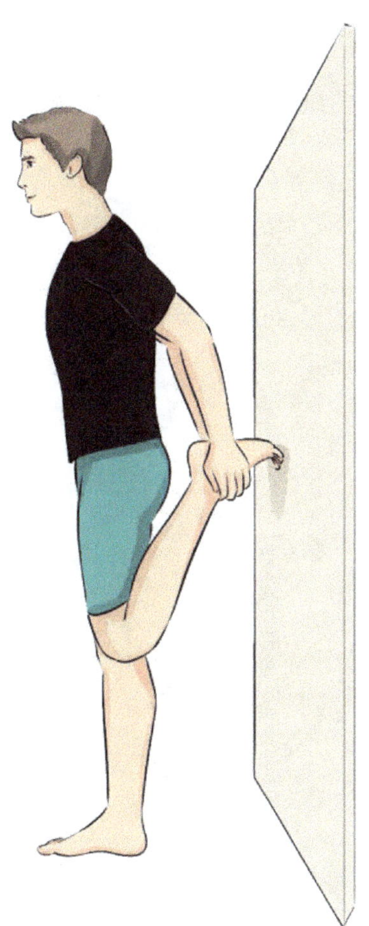

Instructions

1. Stand facing way from the wall with your feet hip-width apart.
2. Lift your left foot off the ground, bending your knee, and bring your heel toward your buttocks. Hold your left ankle with both hands.
3. Place your toes against the wall for support.
4. Find a distance that allows you to maintain balance and feel a comfortable stretch in your quadriceps.
5. Hold the stretch for 30 seconds to 1 minute, breathing deeply and focusing on relaxing into the stretch.
6. Gently release the stretch by lowering your foot back to the ground. Switch sides and repeat the stretch with your right leg.
7. Perform 2 sets of 6 reps on each leg.

Tips:

- Keep a slight bend in the knee to prevent strain on the joint.

- If balance is challenging, you can place one hand on the wall for additional stability.

- Gradually increase the intensity of the stretch over time and you can eventually balance without the wall!

14 | COW POSE

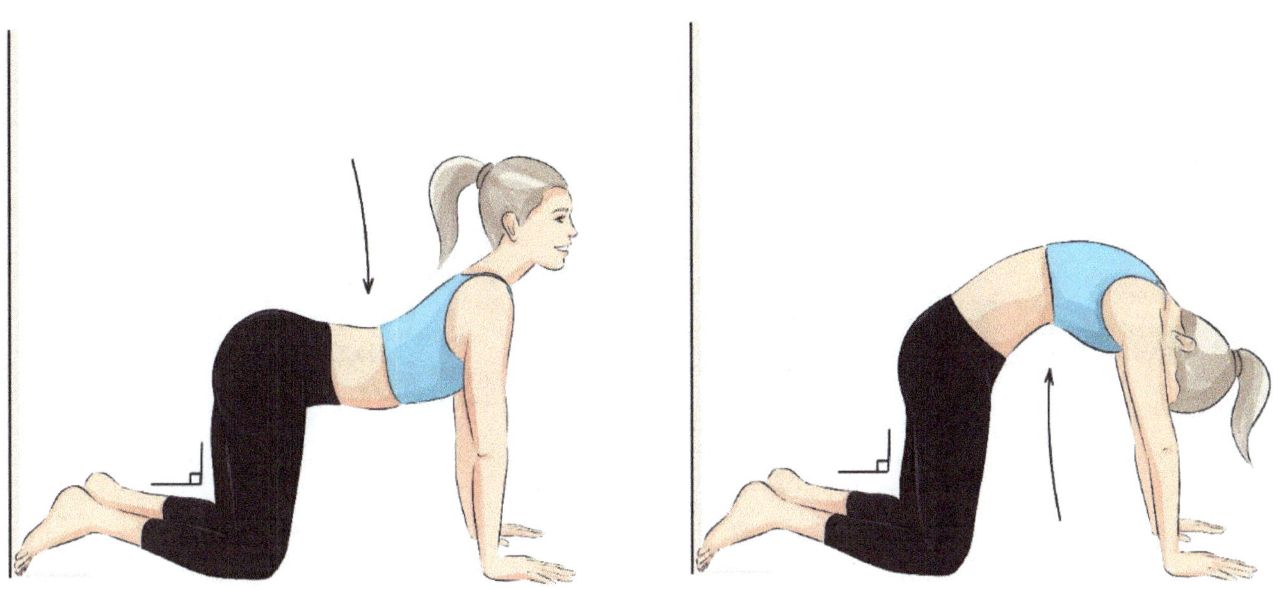

Instructions

1. Begin on your hands and knees in a tabletop position. Ensure that your wrists are directly under your shoulders and your knees are directly under your hips.
2. Check that your spine is in a neutral position, neither arched nor rounded. Keep your head in a neutral position, looking down at the mat.
3. Inhale deeply and smoothly through your nose, preparing for the movement. As you exhale, tilt your pelvis up toward the ceiling, arching your back. Allow your belly to sink toward the floor, creating a concave shape in your spine.
4. Lift your head and tailbone toward the ceiling. Your gaze should be forward or slightly upward, but avoid straining your neck by dropping your head too far back.
5. Open your chest by broadening your collarbones. Imagine squeezing your shoulder blades together behind you.
6. Hold the Cow Pose for a few breaths, focusing on the expansion of your chest and the stretch along your spine.
7. Perform the Cow Pose for 10 reps.

Tips:

*   Coordinate each movement with either an inhalation or an exhalation.
*   If you have any wrist issues, you can come on to your fists or use a yoga wedge to reduce the pressure on your wrists.

15 | ROLL-UP

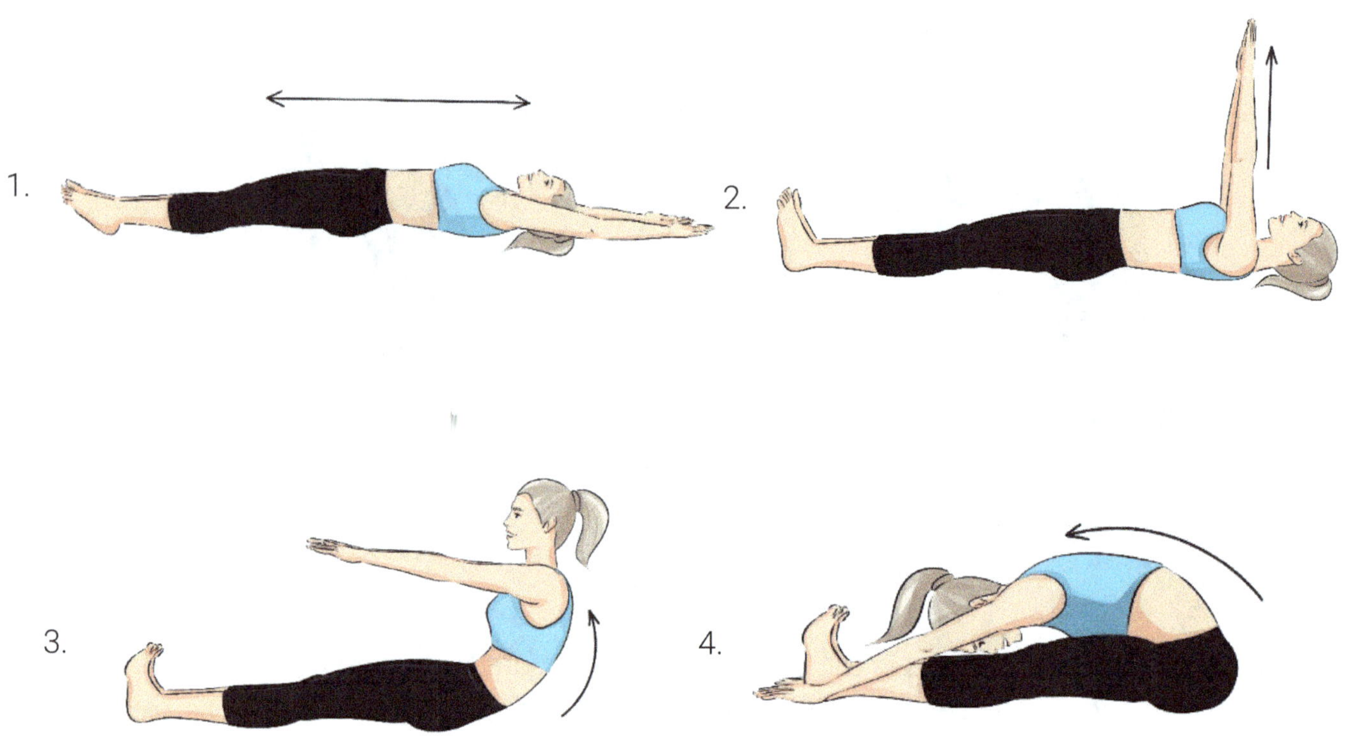

Instructions

1. Begin by lying on your back on a mat with your legs extended and your arms reaching overhead. Your legs should be together. Keep your arms in line with your ears throughout.
2. Inhale to prepare for the movement. Lengthen your spine along the mat and engage your abdominal muscles.
3. As you exhale, begin to lift your spine off the mat. Imagine peeling your spine off the mat one vertebra at a time.
4. Continue the movement by reaching your arms forward toward your toes.
5. At the top of the movement, your body should form a shape similar to the letter C, and your abdominals should be deeply engaged.
6. Inhale to prepare for the descent. As you exhale, slowly and with control, begin to roll your spine back down to the mat one vertebra at a time.
7. Once your entire spine is back on the mat, inhale and extend your arms overhead, returning to the starting position.
8. Perform 8–10 reps of the Roll-Up, maintaining a smooth and controlled movement throughout.

Tips:

- If you find it challenging to Roll-up smoothly, you can modify the exercise by bending your knees slightly or by placing a small towel or cushion under your lower back for support.

- Focus on engaging your core muscles throughout the entire exercise to protect your lower back.

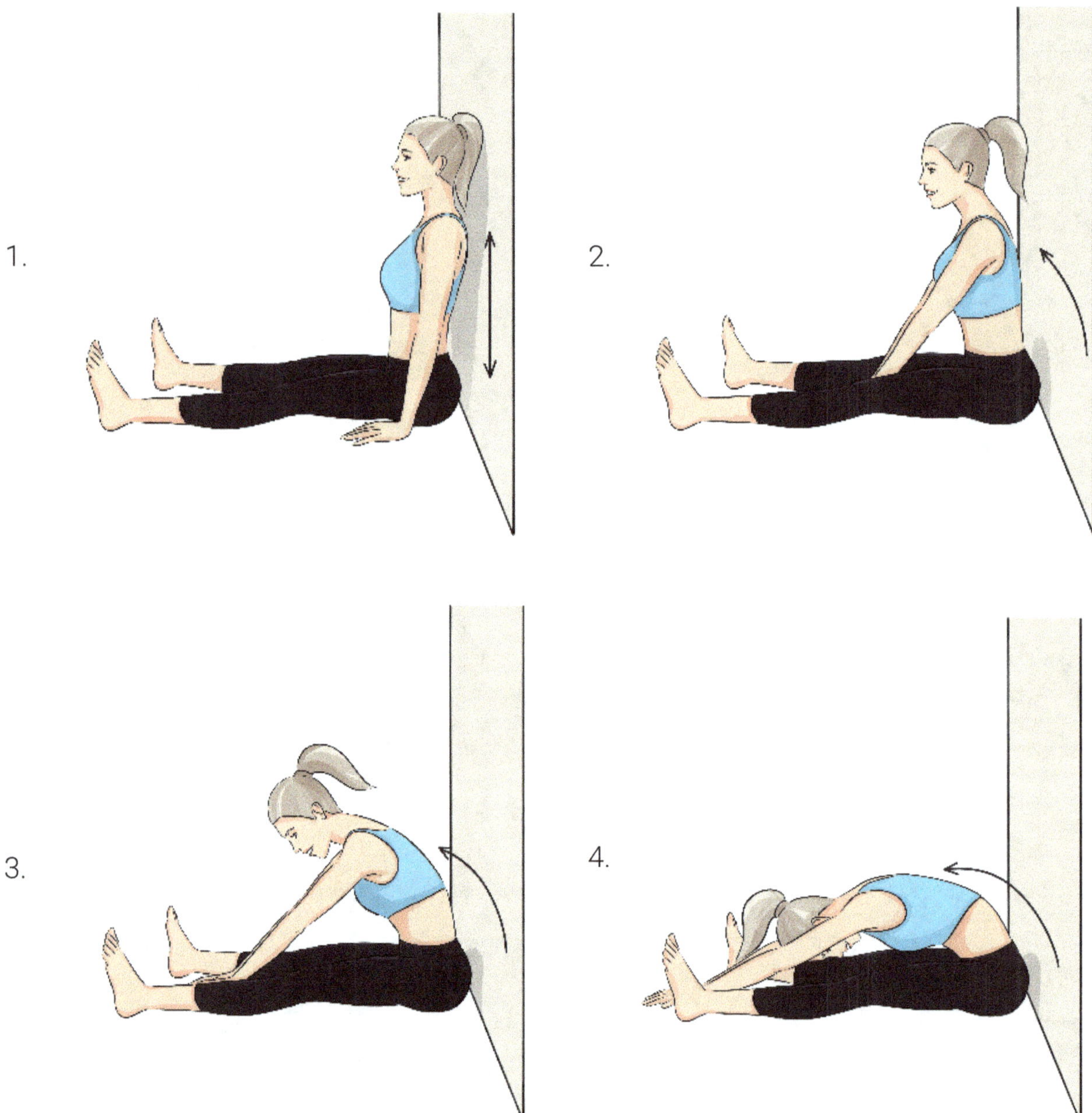

Instructions

1. Sit on a mat with your legs extended straight in front of you. Sit tall with your spine in a neutral position, shoulders relaxed, and arms extended straight out in front of you at shoulder height.
2. Inhale deeply through your nose, expanding your rib cage and engaging your core. As you exhale through your mouth, tuck your chin to your chest and your spine forward, one vertebra at a time.
3. Imagine reaching the crown of your head forward as you move, creating length in your spine. Throughout the movement, keep your arms parallel to the floor, reaching straight forward. Maintain a slight bend in your elbows to avoid locking them.

4. Continue rounding your back until you feel a stretch along your spine and the back of your legs. The goal is to create a "C-curve" shape with your spine.
5. If comfortable, reach your hands toward your toes, keeping your spine rounded.
6. Inhale to prepare to return to the starting position. As you exhale, start to stack your spine back up, vertebra by vertebra.
7. Once you're back in the starting position, sit tall with your shoulders over your hips and your spine in a neutral alignment.
8. Perform 10 reps.

Tips:

- Keep your shoulders relaxed and down, avoiding tension in the neck and upper traps.

- If you have tight hamstrings, it's okay to keep a slight bend in your knees during the exercise.

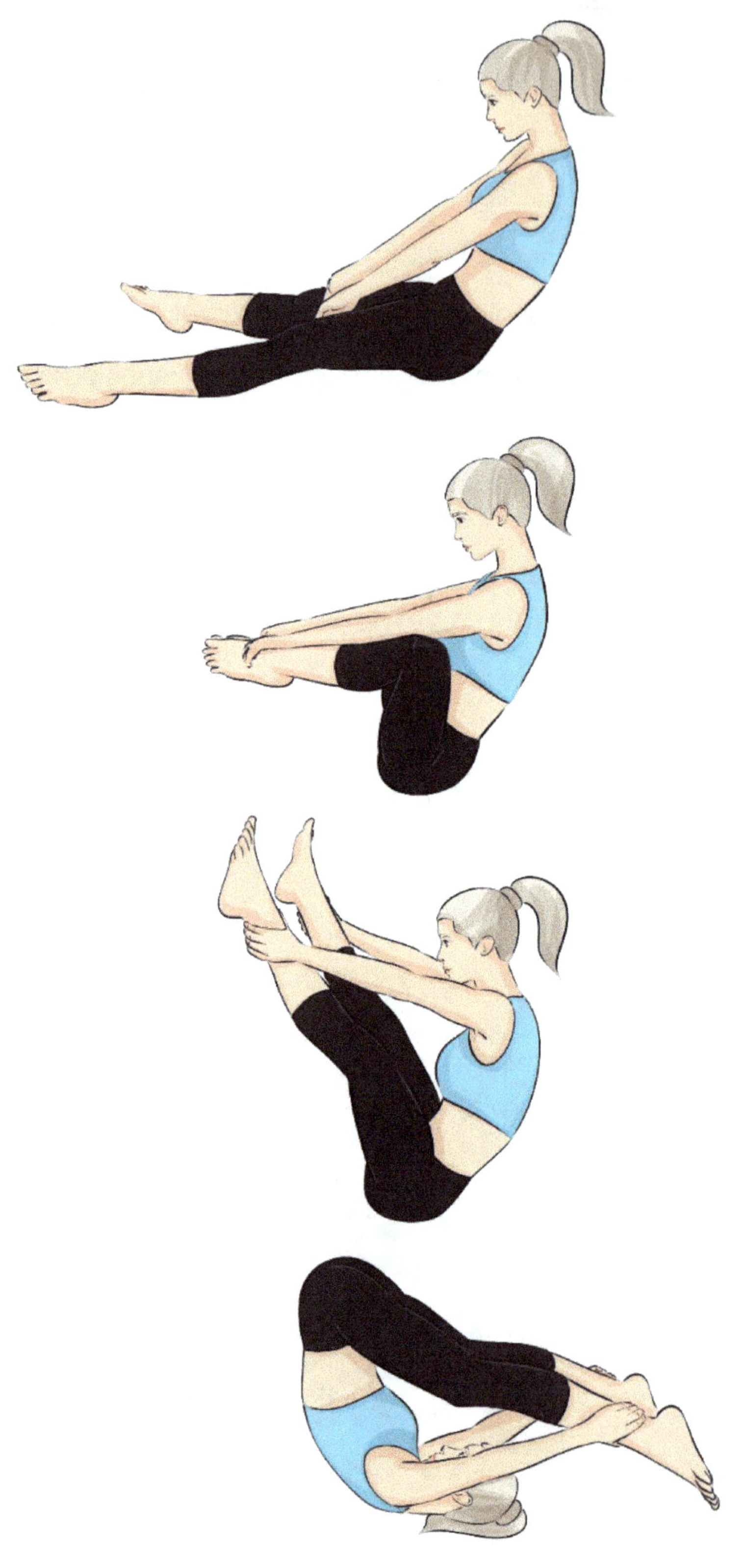

Instructions

1. Sit on a mat with your knees bent and your feet flat on the floor. Hold on to the backs of your thighs with your hands, sitting tall with a straight spine.
2. Inhale to prepare, and as you exhale, open your knees to the sides while keeping your feet together. Your legs will form a diamond shape with the soles of your feet touching.
3. Balancing on your sit bones, engage your core muscles to lift your feet off the mat, bringing your shins parallel to the floor. Your upper body remains upright, forming a V shape with your torso and thighs.
4. Reach your arms forward, parallel to the floor, and hold on to the outsides of your thighs just above your knees. Your hands maintain contact with your thighs throughout the exercise.
5. Inhale deeply, and as you exhale, lean back, rolling onto your sacrum while maintaining the V shape position with your torso and thighs. Keep your feet off the mat.
6. Exhale as you use your core muscles to rock back up to the balanced V-position. Find your balance on your sit bones without letting your feet touch the mat.
7. Continue rocking back and forth, coordinating your breath with the movement. Inhale as you lean back and exhale as you return to the balanced V-position.
8. Repeat the rocking motion for 8 reps. Do 3 sets.

Tips:

- Keep your chest lifted and your shoulders relaxed throughout the exercise.

- If you find it challenging to maintain balance, you can place a small cushion or rolled-up mat under your sacrum for support.

- Focus on using your abdominal muscles to control the rocking motion.

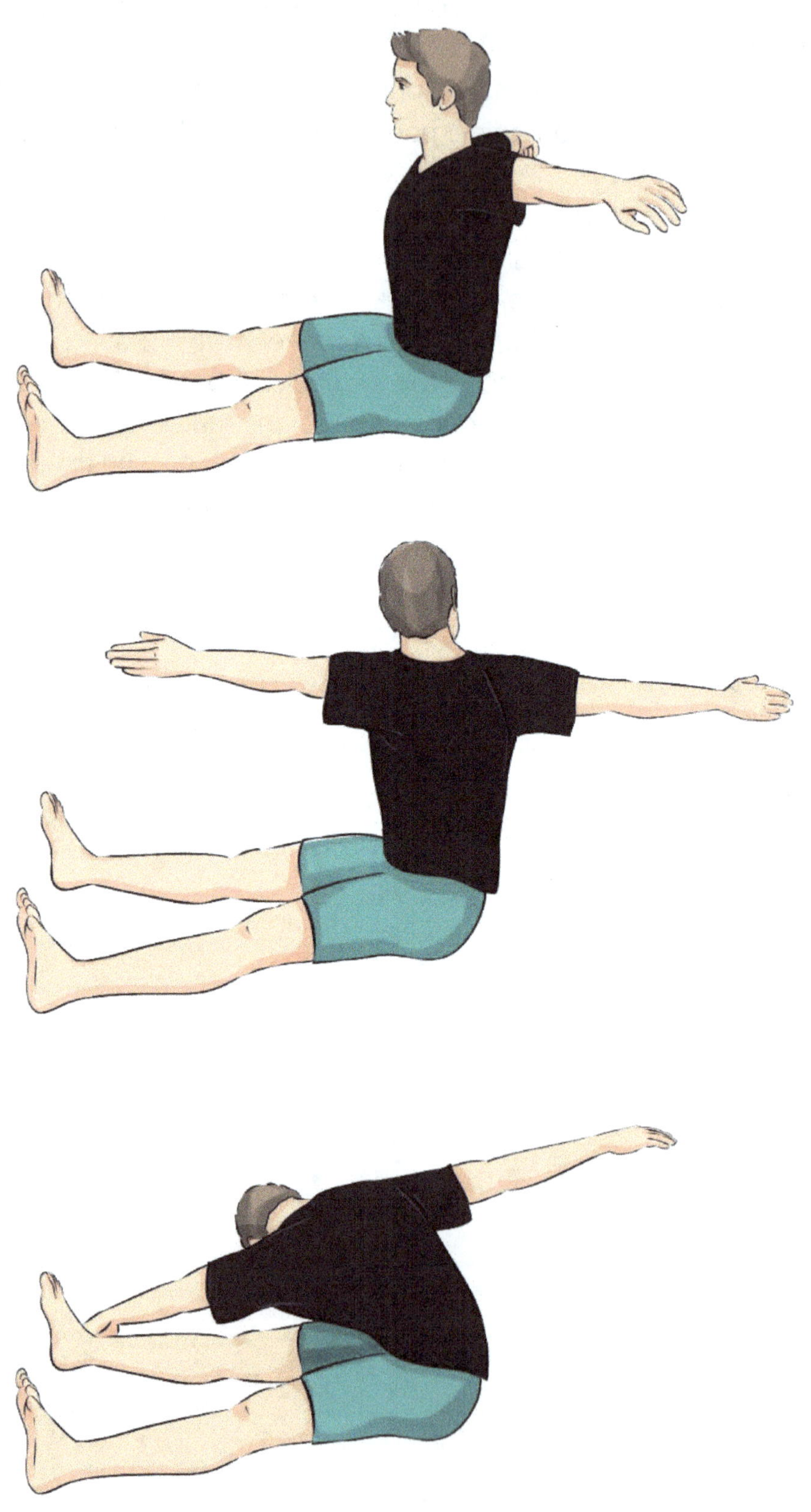

Instructions

1. Begin by sitting on a mat with your legs extended straight in front of you. Open your legs slightly wider than hip-width apart. Sit tall with a straight spine, engaging your core muscles.
2. Extend your arms out to the sides, parallel to the floor. Your arms should be in line with your shoulders, forming a T shape.
3. Inhale deeply through your nose. As you exhale, rotate your torso to the right, reaching your left hand toward your right foot. Your right arm reaches behind you, and your gaze follows your right hand.
4. As you rotate, lead with your pinky finger, reaching toward the baby toe of your right foot. Keep your spine long and avoid rounding your back.
5. Ensure that your hips remain squared to the front throughout the movement. Avoid letting one hip lift higher than the other.
6. Flex your left foot, reaching through the heel to engage the back of the leg. Inhale to come back to the center, returning to the starting position with arms extended to the sides.
7. Do the same actions for the left leg and continue alternating from side to side, moving with controlled and fluid movements.
8. Perform 2 sets of 8 reps.

Tips:

- Focus on the rotation coming from your waist and upper back, not just your shoulders.

- Keep your abdominals engaged to support your spine during the rotation.

- Aim to create length through your spine, maintaining good posture throughout the exercise.

19 | DOWNWARD DOG

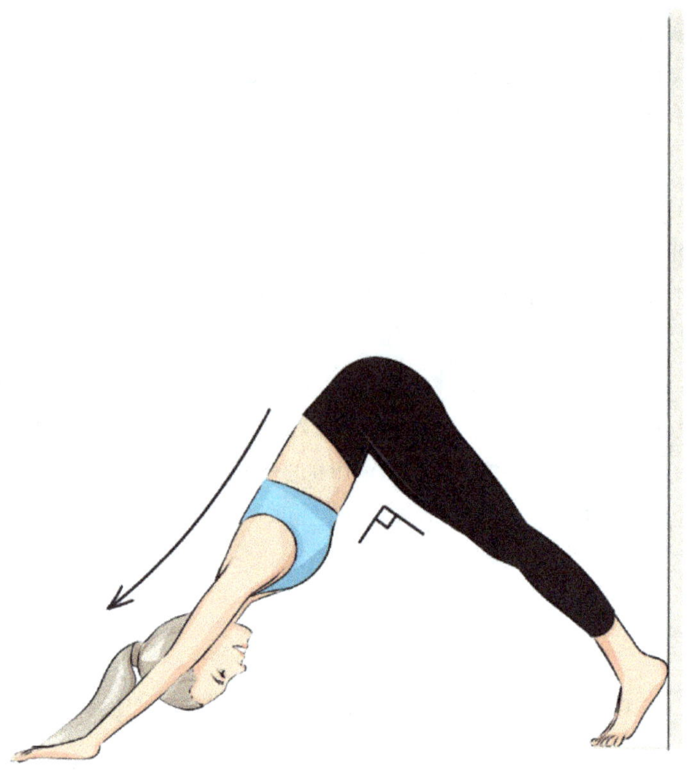

Instructions:

1. Begin on your hands and knees in a tabletop position, aligning your wrists under your shoulders and your knees under your hips.
2. Plant your hands firmly on the mat with your fingers spread wide. Your middle fingers should point directly forward. Tuck your toes under, lifting your knees off the mat.
3. Exhale and begin to straighten your legs, lifting your hips toward the ceiling. Your body will form an inverted V shape.
4. Focus on lengthening your spine by reaching your tailbone toward the ceiling and pressing your chest toward your thighs. Your ears should be in line with your upper arms.
5. To avoid hyperextension, maintain a slight bend in your knees.
6. Engage your core.
7. Allow your head to hang freely between your arms. Avoid tensing your neck. If needed, shake your head gently from side to side to release tension. Draw your shoulder blades down your back, opening your chest and broadening your upper back.
8. Take deep breaths in and out through your nose. Expand your rib cage with each inhale and elongate your spine with each exhale.
9. Hold the Downward Dog for 30 seconds to 1 minute or longer.
10. Perform 2 sets of 10 reps.

Tips:

- Keep your knees slightly bent if you have tight hamstrings.

- Experiment with the width of your hands and the distance between your feet to find a comfortable and stable position.

Strength Exercises

Strength training plays a crucial role in enhancing balance, stability, and overall functional fitness, especially for seniors.

Strength training helps build and maintain muscle strength and endurance. Stronger muscles are better equipped to support the body's weight and provide stability during various activities.

Strengthening the muscles around the joints contributes to joint stability. This is particularly important for the ankles, knees, and hips, which are key areas for maintaining balance.

Sarcopenia is the age-related loss of muscle mass and strength. Strength training is an effective way to counteract this natural process and preserve muscle mass, contributing to improved balance and stability.

20 | WALL SIT WITH TAI CHI ARM RAISES

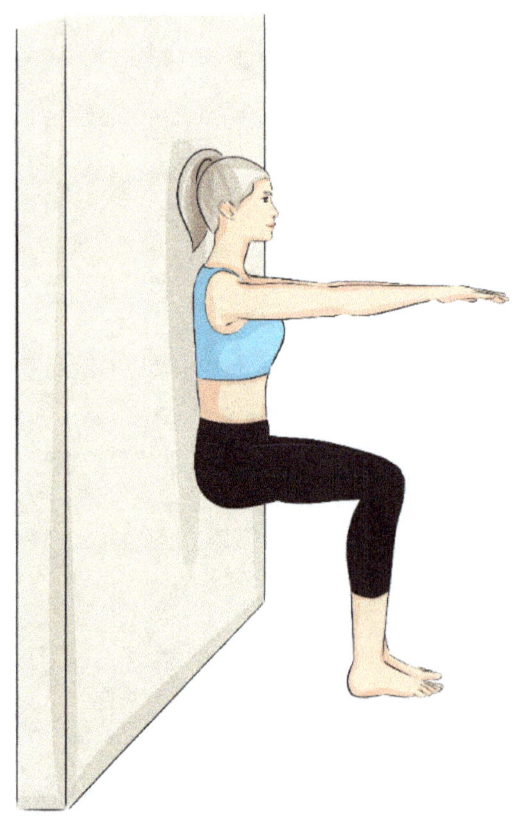

Instructions

1. Stand with your back against a wall, and then slowly walk your feet forward, allowing your spine to slide down the wall. Keep your feet hip-width apart.

2. Bend your knees and lower your body into a sitting position against the wall. Ensure your knees are directly above your ankles, forming a 90-degree angle with your thighs parallel to the floor.
3. Begin the Tai Chi arm raises by inhaling and lifting your arms in front of you. Keep your palms facing down and allow your arms to float up as if they are moving through water.
4. Continue raising your arms until they are at shoulder height, reaching forward with your fingertips. Maintain a gentle and controlled pace, focusing on the smoothness of the movement.
5. Exhale as you slowly lower your arms back down to your starting position.
6. Repeat the Tai Chi arm raises 10–15 times, coordinating the movement with your breath.

Tips:

- Keep your back firmly against the wall throughout the exercise to ensure proper alignment and engagement of the leg muscles.

- Control the descent into the wall sit position, avoiding a rapid drop.

- Focus on the quality of the arm movements, emphasizing the fluid and controlled nature inspired by tai chi.

21 | SIDE STEPS (LEFT AND RIGHT)

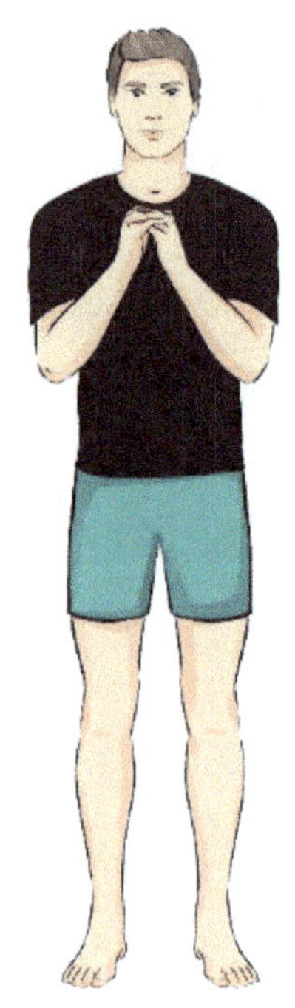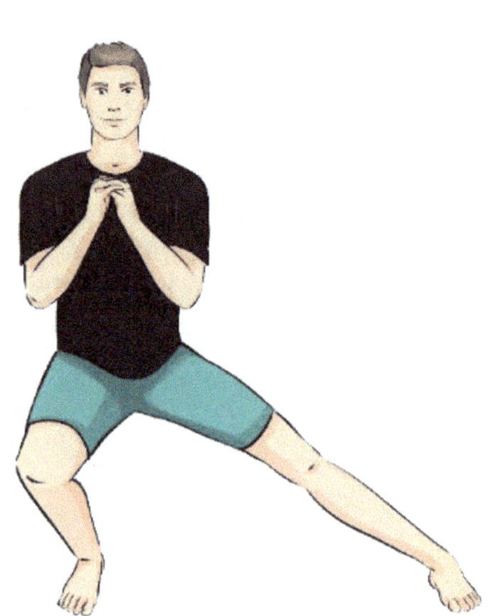

Instructions

1. Stand with your feet hip-width apart and keep your posture upright with your shoulders back and your core engaged. Bend your knees slightly.
2. Place your hands on your hips for added stability.
3. Take a step to the right with your right foot, ensuring that your feet remain parallel. Your left foot follows to meet your right foot. Maintain a slight bend in the knees.
4. Keep your body low to the ground in a slight squat position. This engages the muscles in your thighs and hips.
5. Repeat the same movement, but this time, step to the left with your left foot, followed by your right foot.
6. Continue alternating side steps to the right and left.
7. Perform side steps for 30 seconds. Do 3 sets.

Tip:

- Maintain a slow and controlled pace to maximize muscle engagement and minimize the risk of injury.

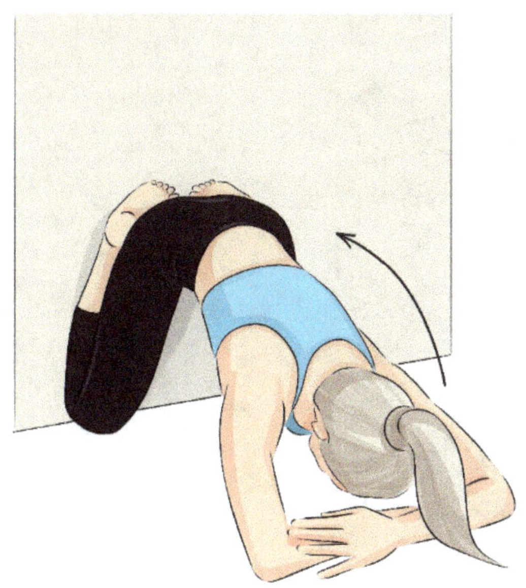 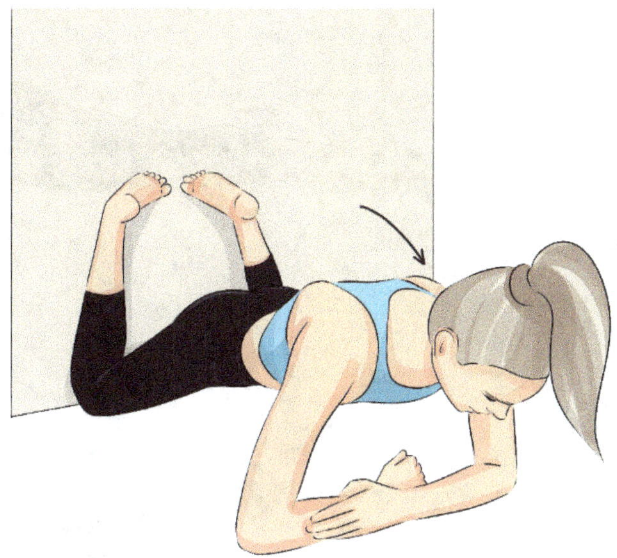

Instructions

1. Stand facing a wall, with your feet hip-width apart. Your toes should be about a foot away from the wall.
2. Lean forward and place your hands on the wall at shoulder height, spreading your fingers wide for stability. Your hands should be aligned with your shoulders.
3. Walk your feet back, stepping away from the wall. As you move your feet back, your body will incline forward, and your torso will start to approach a horizontal position.
4. Engage your core muscles, drawing your navel toward your spine. This is the starting position for the wall-assisted half-body plank.
5. Your body should form a straight line from your head to your heels. Avoid sagging or arching your back. Focus on keeping your body in a plank position.
6. Bend your elbows slightly, bringing your upper body closer to the wall. Your elbows should point backward, not outward. This position engages the muscles in your chest, shoulders, and triceps.
7. Start with a 30-second hold and gradually increase the time as you build strength.
8. Do 2 sets.

Tip:

- If needed, reduce the incline by stepping closer to the wall.

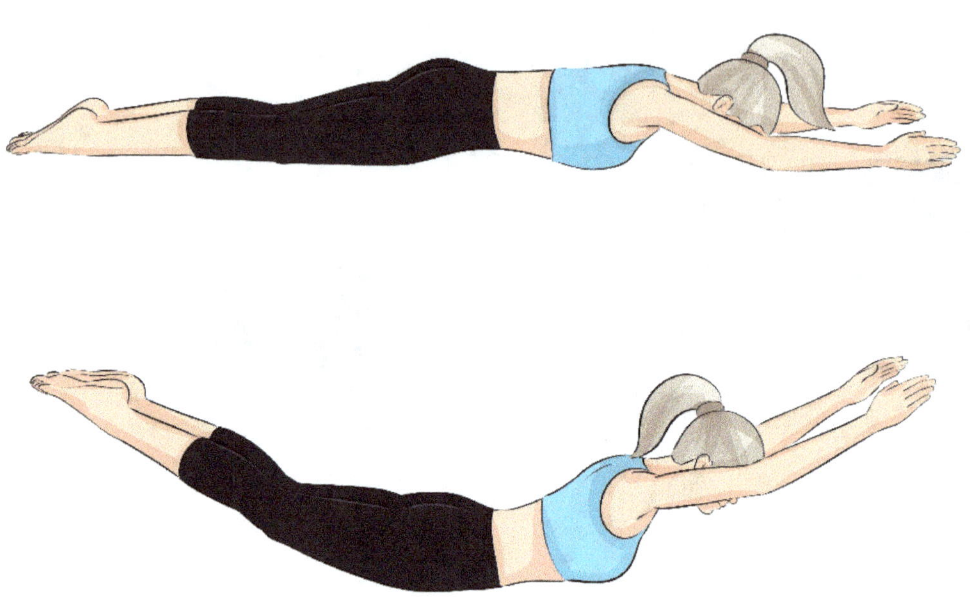

Instructions

1. Lie face down and extend your arms straight in front of you, parallel to the floor. Your legs should be fully extended with your toes pointing away from you.
2. Inhale and simultaneously lift your arms, chest, and legs off the ground. Aim to lift your thighs and chest as high as comfortably possible, creating a gentle curve in your back.
3. At the top of the movement, squeeze your glutes (buttocks) to engage the muscles in your lower back and lift your legs higher.
4. Hold the lifted position for a moment, feeling the contraction in your lower back and glutes. Focus on maintaining good form and a straight line from your head to your toes.
5. Exhale and gently lower your arms, chest, and legs back to the starting position.
6. Perform 2 sets of 10 reps.

Tip:

- Focus on the quality of the movement rather than speed. Lift and lower with control to engage the targeted muscles effectively.

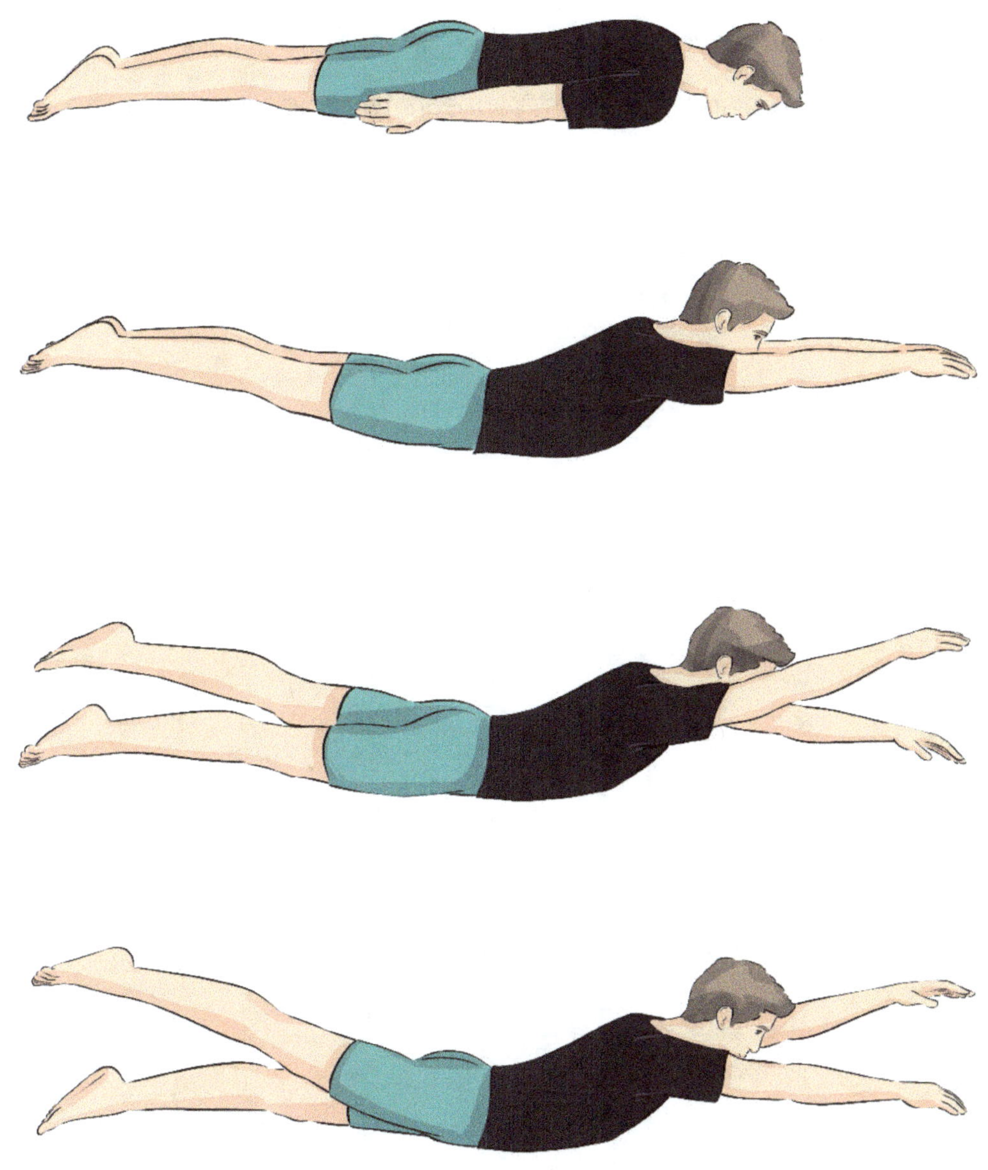

Instructions

1. Lie face down with your arms extended in front of you and your legs fully extended behind you. Ensure your body is in a straight line from your head to your heels.
2. Inhale as you lift your right arm and left leg off the mat simultaneously. Keep your limbs straight and avoid arching your back excessively.
3. Exhale as you lower your right arm and left leg back to the mat and simultaneously lift your left arm and right leg.

4. As you lift your arms and legs, engage your core muscles to lift your chest slightly off the mat.
5. Coordinate the movement of your arms and legs with your breath. Inhale as you lift, and exhale as you lower. Focus on creating a flowing and controlled motion.
6. Perform the Swimming exercise for 2 sets of 30 seconds to 1 minute.

Tips:

- Focus on the quality of the movement rather than speed.

- Keep your shoulders relaxed and away from your ears to avoid tension in the neck and upper traps.

25 | OPPOSITE ARM AND LEG RAISE

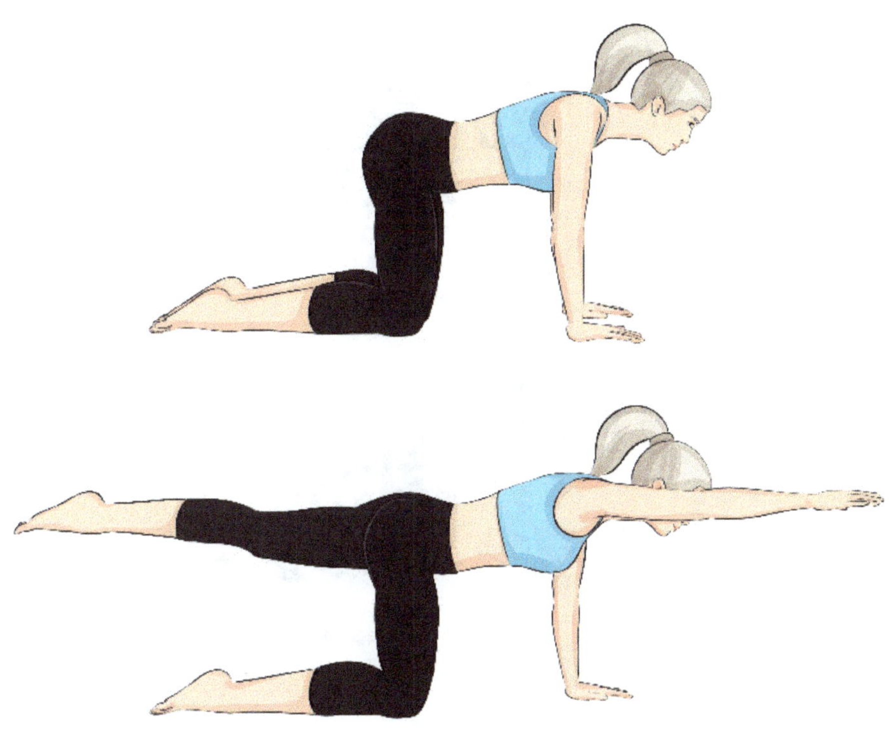

Instructions

1. Begin on your hands and knees in a tabletop position. Ensure your wrists are under your shoulders and your knees are under your hips.
2. Draw your navel toward your spine. This stabilizes your spine and helps maintain a neutral position.
3. Inhale as you extend your right arm forward, reaching it straight out in front of you. Keep your arm in line with your ear.
4. Simultaneously extend your left leg straight back behind you. Aim to create a straight line from your fingertips to your toes. Avoid lifting your leg too high or arching your back. Keep your hips parallel to the floor.
5. Hold the extended position for a moment, focusing on keeping your body stable.
6. Exhale as you lower your right arm and left leg back to the starting tabletop position.
7. Do 2 sets of 10 reps.

Tip:

*   Keep your movements controlled and avoid any sudden or jerky motions to prevent strain on your lower back.

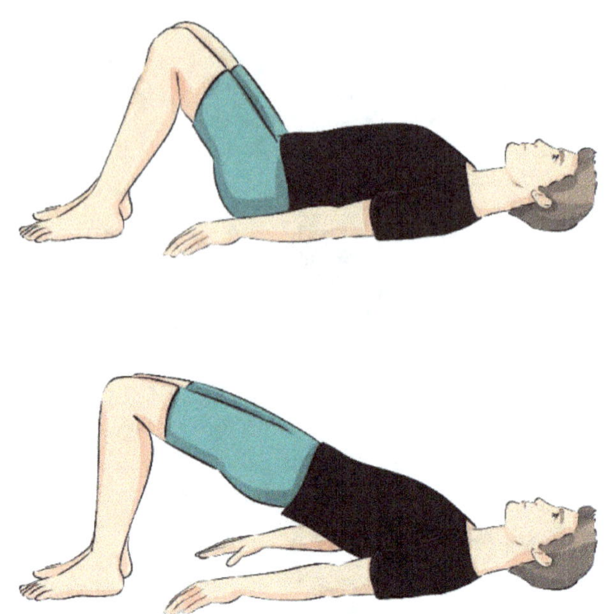

Instructions

1. Lie on your back with your knees bent and your feet flat on the floor. Ensure that your feet are hip-width apart and parallel.
2. Place your arms by your sides, with your palms facing down. Your arms should be close to your body.
3. Activate your core muscles by drawing your navel toward your spine.
4. Inhale and press through your heels, lifting your hips toward the ceiling. Focus on lifting your hips by engaging your glutes and hamstrings, not by arching your lower back.
5. At the top of the bridge, squeeze your glutes to maximize the activation of your posterior chain.
6. Hold the bridge position at the top for 2 seconds, maintaining engagement in your glutes and core.
7. Exhale as you lower your hips back down to the mat in a controlled manner. Avoid letting your hips drop too quickly.
8. Perform 2 sets of 10 reps.

Tips:

- Keep your knees aligned with your feet and avoid letting them collapse inward during the movement.

- Focus on the quality of the movement rather than lifting your hips too high.

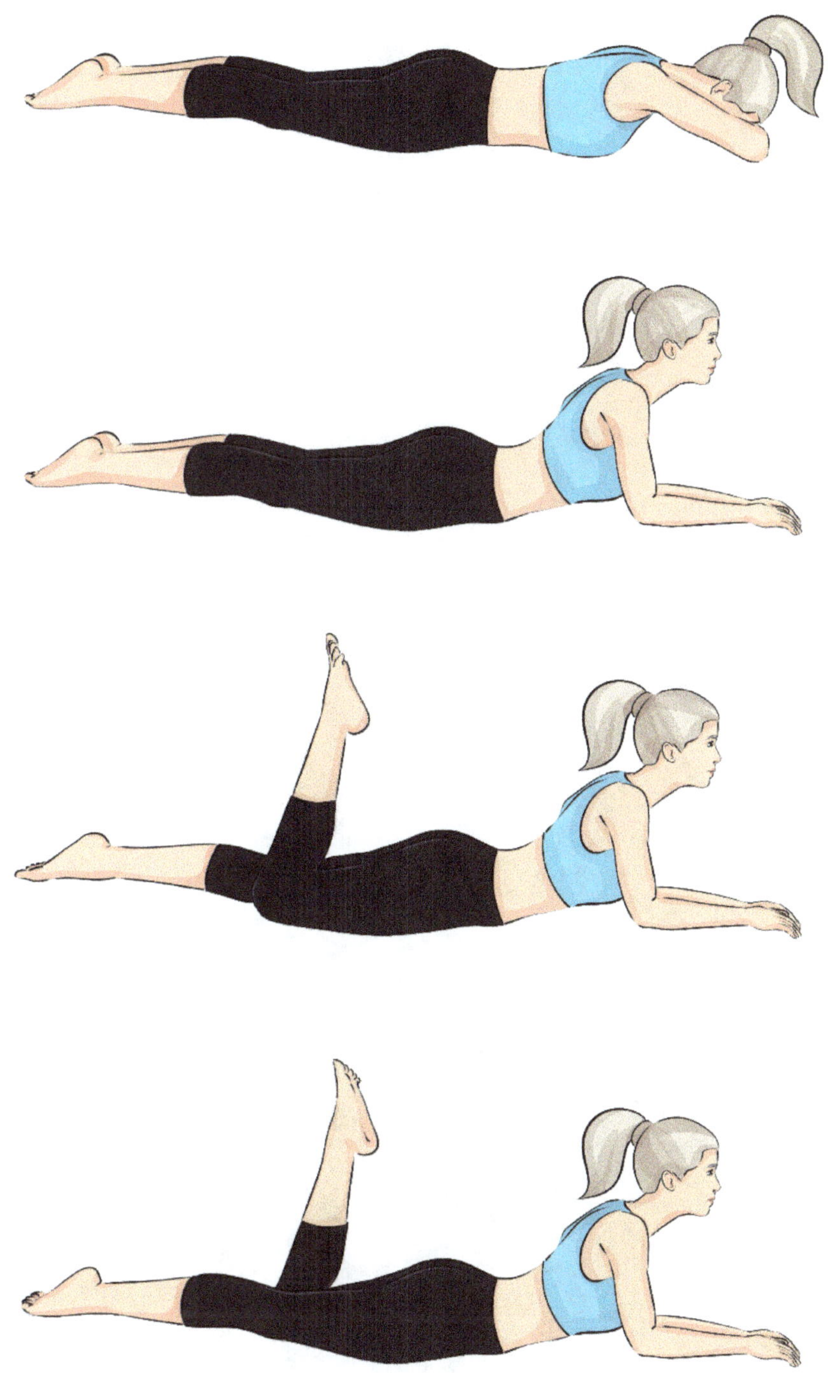

Instructions

1. Lie face down with your legs extended straight and your forehead resting on the mat. Your arms should be positioned alongside your body, palms facing down.
2. Inhale as you bend your right leg, bringing your heel toward your buttocks. The knee remains close to the mat, forming a 90-degree angle with your thigh.

3. Exhale and kick your right leg out straight, engaging your hamstring and glutes. Keep the kick controlled, and avoid lifting your thigh off the mat.
4. Point your toes during the kick to create length in your leg.
5. Inhale as you lower your right leg back to the starting position, bending the knee again.
6. Repeat on the other leg.
7. Do 3 sets of 12 reps on each leg.

Tip:

- Keep your movements controlled to engage the targeted muscles effectively and avoid straining your lower back.

28 | THE CONTROL BALANCE

This can be difficult if you have back or pelvic pain so please consult a Pilates instructor if you are unsure. Use the wall to find safety and if you lose balance.

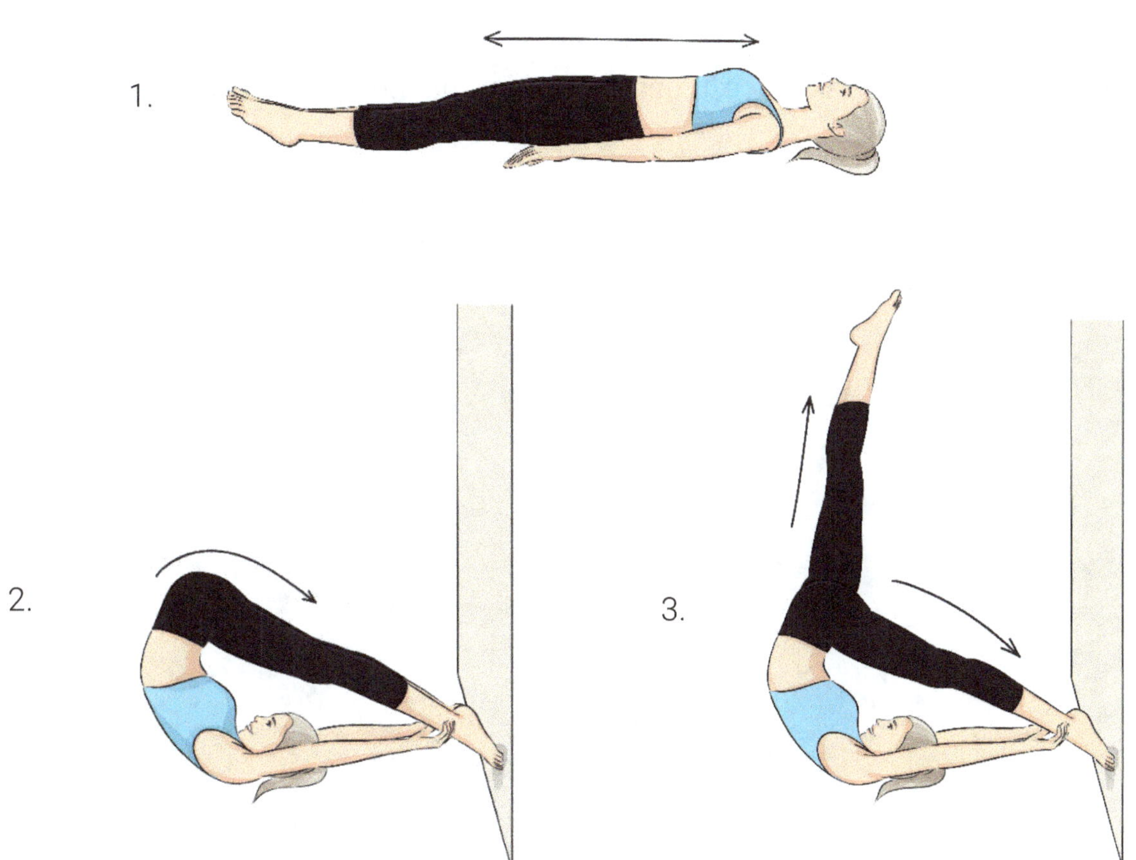

Instructions

1. Begin by sitting on the floor with your knees bent and your feet flat. Place your hands behind you, fingers pointing backward, and lift your hips into a reverse tabletop position.
2. Extend your right leg straight up toward the ceiling while keeping your left foot on the mat. Your body should now form an inverted L shape.
3. Inhale and extend your left leg straight, lifting it toward the ceiling. Both legs should be extended, creating a straight line from your shoulders through your hips to your toes.
4. Shift your weight onto your hands and lift your hips, bringing your torso more perpendicular to the mat.
5. Engage your core muscles to find balance in the inverted position. Keep your shoulders down, away from your ears, and your neck in a neutral position.
6. Keep both legs straight and energized. Point your toes to create length in your legs. Control the balance by using your core muscles. Avoid rocking or swinging, and focus on stabilizing your body.

7. Hold the Control Balance for a few breaths, maintaining stability with steady inhalations and exhalations.
8. To release from the Control Balance, lower your legs with control back to the mat, returning to the reverse tabletop position.
9. Do 2 sets of 12 reps on each leg.

Repeat on the other side.

Tip:

- If you're new to the Control Balance, practice with another person nearby or near a sturdy surface to assist with balance.

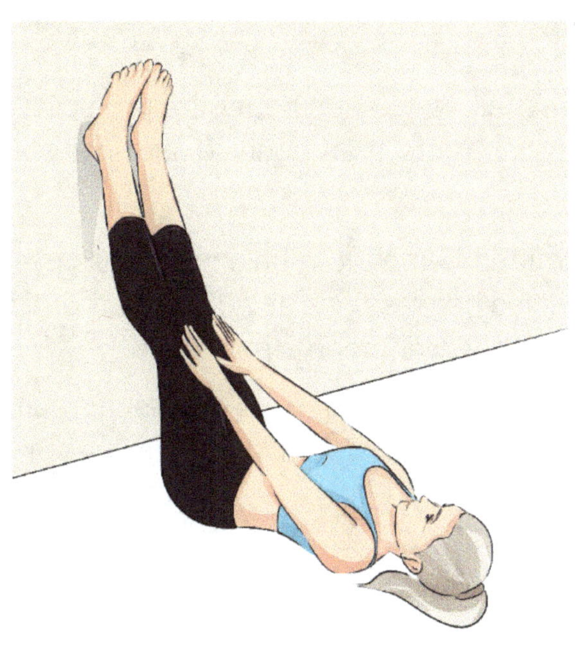 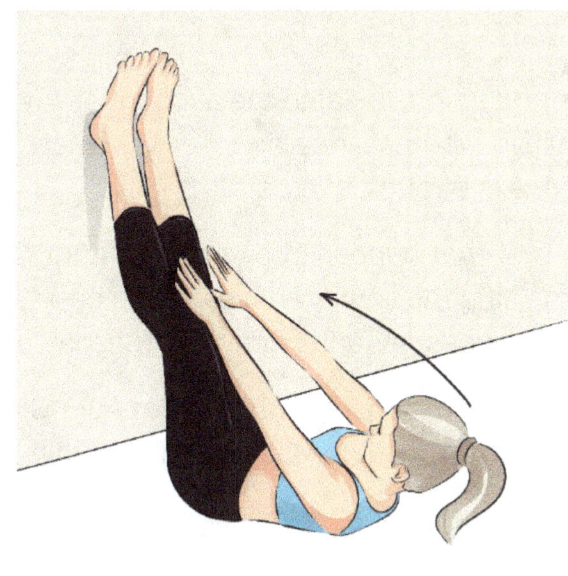

Instructions

1. Lie on your back with your legs fully extended and your arms reaching overhead. Your body should be in a straight line.
2. Inhale as you lift your arms off the floor and reach them toward the ceiling. Your arms should stay in line with your ears.
3. Exhale and lift your upper body off the floor, reaching your hands toward your toes. Imagine bringing your rib cage toward your pelvis.
4. Maintain straight legs throughout the movement. Engage your quadriceps to keep your legs extended.
5. Aim to touch your toes with your hands. If you can't reach your toes, that's okay; the goal is to lift and reach toward them.
6. Inhale as you lower your upper body back down to the mat with control. Keep your lower back in contact with the mat throughout the descent.
7. Perform 2 sets of 10 reps. Gradually increase the number of reps as you build strength.

Tips:

- Keep your neck in a neutral position by looking toward the ceiling during the movement. Avoid pulling on your neck with your hands.

- If you find it challenging to keep your legs straight, you can slightly bend your knees.

Start Today, Start Now

In the introduction, I related the account of my Aunt Clara's fall. Now, she's better than she ever was. Her positive vibe has returned, her lower body strength has more than doubled, and her balance confidence is through the roof.

But none of that happened by chance. Aunt Clara committed herself to a balance fitness exercise program using the very exercises in this book. She scheduled her sessions at 7:30 every morning on Monday, Wednesday, and Friday. On Tuesday and Thursday, she went for a 2-mile walk.

I'd love for you to take inspiration from Aunt Clara. Don't be one of those people who read a self-help book, gathers all the knowledge, and then fails to put it into action.

Your body deserves better than that!

Set a date to begin your balance exercise program, and then commit to it. I recommend doing your workouts three times per week on alternate days and then doing some light cardio, such as a walk, on your days off, just like Aunt Clara does.

Here's a recap of how to structure your workouts:

- Choose 3 Warm-up exercises to begin your workout.
- Choose 3 exercises from the Awareness in Movement section.
- Choose 3 exercises from the Alignment section.
- Choose 3 exercises from the Flexibility section.
- Choose 3 exercises from the Strength section.

As you engage in these balance exercises, by the fifth or sixth session, you will start to feel a noticeable improvement in your stability and coordination. By the tenth session, you'll likely experience enhanced strength and confidence in your movements. As you reach the twentieth session, incorporating these exercises will become second nature, seamlessly fitting into your routine.

Your Free Gift

Before we part ways, remember your purchase of this book comes with a bonus: The Ultimate Kegels Guide. It works for both men and women!

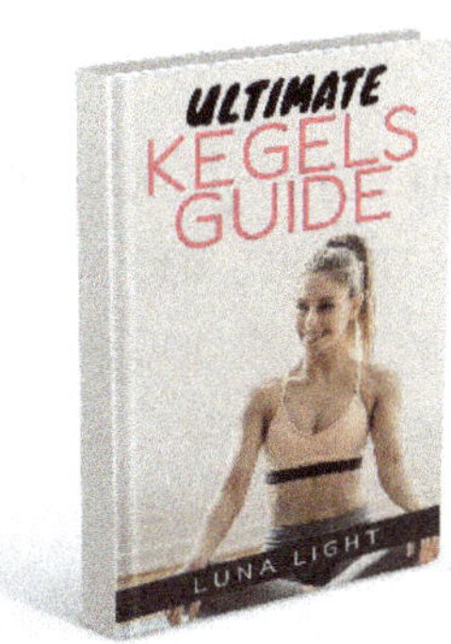

You may have heard of Kegels before... but unfortunately, there is widespread misinformation about hold time, number of repetitions and how to actually perform the contractions that do more bad than good.

When done right, Kegels are a powerful way to build endurance, increase strength in your core and enhance your sex life. The Kegels exercise we created comes directly from Tim Sawyer, a top physical therapist who worked with doctors at Stanford University2 to develop rehabilitation programs.

This exact Kegels exercise has helped tremendously in improving my pelvic floor tone, enhancing my sex life, and developing a strong core.

All you have to do is go to wallpilates.org to download it for free. Alternatively, scan the QR code below:

---

[2] Dr. Wise and Dr. Anderson authored A Headache in the Pelvis: A New Understanding and Treatment for Chronic Pelvic Pain Syndromes and consulted Tim as the main physical therapist for their treatments.

Thank You

My name is Luna, and it has been my pleasure to serve you. You could have picked from dozens of other books, but you took a chance and chose this one. So, thank you for investing in yourself and making it to the end!

Before we say goodbye, one question: If you enjoyed this book, would you consider leaving a review? A review is the easiest and best way to support the work of independent authors like me. Your feedback will help us continue writing the types of books that will help you and others in the journey to good health.

You can leave a review here in 15 seconds:

Luna's Books On Amazon

To your happiness and health,
— Luna Light